Brigitte Gaertner

Powerful Feng Shui Balancing Tools

Minor Accents with Major Effects
The Mysterious Magic of
Crystals, Chimes, Spirals, and Much More for Your Magnificent Feng Shui Home

Translated by Christine M. Grimm

ARCANA PUBLISHING

Graphic Art Information:
Kuhn Grafik: pg. 8, 9
Peter Ehrhardt: pg. 22 (Dragon)
Samuel Kwok: All calligraphy except:
Wang Ning: pg. 35, 72, 89
Schneelöwe: pg. 41, 45

Photography Information:
Schneelöwe: pg. 28, 46, 47
Ulrich Geiser: pg. 56, 60 (below)
Ulla Mayer-Raichle: pg. 58
PRIMAVERA LIFE GmbH: pg. 29 ("Avalon" room fountain),
pg. 69 (incense), pg. 85 (feng shui gift set)
L. A. Matzing-Diethelm Travel: pg. 64 (below)

First English Edition 2000
© by Arcana Publishing
an imprint of Lotus Brands, Inc.
P.O. Box 325
Twin Lakes, WI 53181, USA
Published in cooperation
with Schneelöwe Verlagsberatung, Federal Republic of Germany
© 1999 by Windpferd Verlagsgesellschaft mbH, Aitrang, Germany
All rights reserved
Translated by Christine M. Grimm
Cover design by Kuhn Graphik und Buchdesign, Zürich, Switzerland
using a photo by Ulla Mayer-Raichle

ISBN 0-910261-20-2

Printed in Germany

Table of Contents

Preface

The Theory of Happy Rooms

Imagine that the rooms in your apartment or house have a voice and could speak with you.

What are the things that your kitchen, bathroom, entrance hall, living room, bedroom, and storeroom would say to you and tell you? They would certainly thank you for the laughter and life that takes place within their walls; for keeping them clean, taking care of them, and using them; for lovingly decorating and furnishing them. Yet, some of the rooms—such as the storeroom and entrance hall—may also complain about boredom or careless treatment. Either consciously or unconsciously, we are probably already aware of most of the individual rooms' wishes. However, our rooms cannot speak— and ignoring them is so simple.

But sometimes, our own inner voice speaks for the rooms. Then we get caught up in spring cleaning, furnishing fever, or the desire to redecorate.

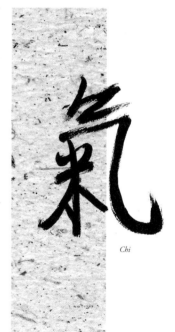

Chi

Every room, every space, no matter how small the apartment may be, would like to be more and can be more than just a rented or purchased surface that has a mailbox with our nameplate standing in front of it. The more we do for our rooms and give them love and care, the more they can give back to us. This cosmic law applies not only to living beings—it stands above everything. When we let our rooms awaken through the knowledge of feng shui, we experience the wonderful enchantment of the private world we live in and how it becomes a place of power. The way in which we furnish our entire living space and how we do this, as well as the zones where we rest or are active, determine the width of our personal path of happiness. When the harmonious aura of a room pampers us with vitality like a source of fresh energy, inspiring the mind and nourishing the soul, then we blossom. Powers awaken within us that had been previously concealed from our inner eyes.

A happy room is loved, cared for, and kept in good condition by its human being so that it can give warmth, light, a sense of security, abundance, inspiration, joy, and power back to that person.

An Absolute Coincidence

In my courses and consultations, people tell me time and again that renting exactly the apartment or house they now have was "an absolute coincidence." Sometimes the conclusion of rental contracts includes very astonishing stories. Every apartment or house—no matter whether it is full of nooks and crannies, linear, spacious, cozy, practical, or whatever else—has its own aura. Even the fact that areas are missing is felt to be extremely charming on the conscious or unconscious level because the "non-existence" is experienced as a very liberating fact when the future occupant sees the dwelling for the first time. The home's floor plan is a mirror of the life situation, in both its good and bad aspects. Many creative minds are magically attracted to stairs that lead downward "into the underground and the depths," while other people experience this living situation as absolutely out of the question.

There are no coincidences—or, in other words: what is suitable for us will come to us quite naturally.

Every home that we have is a mirror of our personality, our goals, our needs, and our life.

The Ideal Floor Plan

If you furnish and orient your apartment or house according to the principles of feng shui, you will very quickly discover that many things make sense in theory but are sometimes impossible to translate into reality. The square or rectangular floor plan cannot simply be created at will in a rented apartment or even a house. Houses require structural remedies that are not always approved or even practicable-plus, this type of renovation also costs a lot of money. In rented apartments, it is absolutely impossible to integrate the missing portion of the floor plan into the occupant's own living space since this usually involves part of the neighboring apartment or the hallway accessible to all residents of the building. It also is not possible to move or alter at will the orientation of the entrance doors in keeping with the four directions. The ideal living situation is therefore actually an exception and compromise solutions are the rule. The more you become involved with feng shui, the more you will come into contact with all types of helpful balancing tools that generally serve to form a bridge between the current state of things and the ideal situation.

Even if the structural aspects of a house are basically correct in every way, the potential of possibilities is naturally far from exhausted. The building with the direction that it faces, its inner divisions, and the existing flow of energy is one of the aspects. However, every house has people living in it and this fact should not be forgotten when dealing with feng shui. Even if a building existed long before we moved into it and will even outlive us, it can only truly be awakened to life by the people who live in it.

Small Things—Big Effects

Every culture has its good-luck charms and its symbols. These are usually very specific things, little objects, amulets, and pictorial depictions. However, each culture also has certain "rules" for increasing the sense of well-being. For example, old farmhouses in Germany usually have the tiled stove built at the center so that the heat can radiate like the sun in all directions. This is a classic feng shui rule since all people experience radiant warmth as a pleasure. So it isn't surprising that this "rule" can be found in all cultures. The same applies to the fountain in front of a house and much, much more.

Often, the small things in a home have the biggest effects. Even if two apartments are furnished in almost exactly the same way, one of them may create a warm impression and the other will seem cold and sterile. However, the sense of well-being is not sparked by the number of things in a room but where they are placed and how they are arranged.

The magic word for achieving the ideal living situation is:

Improve and optimize to the maximum degree.

We have a fantastic tool in our hands in the small things that are put to use in a very conscious way. With them, we can create an abundance and apply the force of positive energies. We are familiar with many of these small objects because we have seen them, but often lack the information to know why they are useful and how to employ them. We could almost compare this situation to a visit to the builder's supply store. This store has hundreds of different tools that are all good for some sort of purpose—for the carpenter, the painter, the plumber, the electrician. But we amateurs stand in front of these shelves with a big question mark in our minds. Even though we just wanted to purchase "a plain old screwdriver," this abundance of supply rattles us and we go home with either an entire set of screwdrivers or nothing at all.

Many people feel the same way when confronted with the little feng shui remedies. They have the wish and the will to optimize or change the current situation.

But how? And where? And why?

This book is intended to answer all of these questions and explain the endless abundance of balancing tools and remedies. Then you can also use all of these wonderful and helpful objects for yourself since they are available to you.

Feng shui remedies are almost like elevator switches that only need to be touched very gently. Without much effort on our part, they take us to the upper levels. People who don't know how to operate an elevator have no choice but to use all of their strength and walk up the steps.

The Fu of Feng Shui

The word *Fu* is translated as "luck." Each of us can certainly make good use of luck at any time, and there is certainly no one who doesn't like to be happy. Feng shui is very much concerned with good fortune since the term "luck" has a much

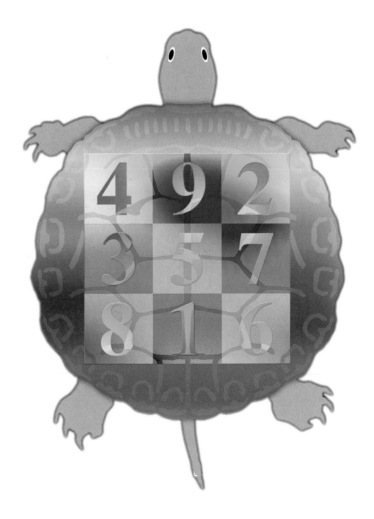

broader meaning and is much more significant in Chinese philosophy than in Western societies. *Pa Kua*, the magical square, contains the philosophy of luck in all 9 sectors:

 The Life Path — Those who have found their path in life are happy because they can see their goal in front of their eyes. This makes the path clear and bright.

 The Relationship — The greatest happiness in life is love.

 The Hierarchy — Those who have found their place in the eternal cycle are free of envy and jealousy. They will be upheld by the strong arms of the family.

 Wealth — Those who harmoniously unite inner and outer wealth have found true happiness.

 Health — The greatest possession and the supreme happiness for us mortal beings is health.

 Helpful Friends — Those who stand by friends in times of need and suffering are rich in help, strength, and support. Those who have the good spirits at their side are never alone. Helpful friends bring back the good luck.

 Joy in Life — Those who laugh and bear the joy and love of life in their hearts are happy, cheerful, and inwardly wealthy.

 Knowledge — Those who are centered like a mountain will receive from a rich spiritual source of good fortune, in which neither doubt nor fears find soil to grow.

Honor — Those who are praised, are honored. Those who receive respect, tolerance, and honor have carried out their deeds to completion and found their own personal, happy *life path*. (The word "life path" corresponds once again with Sector 1, thereby closing the circle.)

9

The Confusion About the Magical Amplifiers of Luck

In a few areas of feng shui, there is "confusion all the way down the line." One of these is that of the remedies and accessories, about which the most abstruse stories are sometimes circulated. The student then relies upon what the course leader has to say about them and what is written in the books. However, there are sometimes completely conflicting statements. Mirrors are one simple example of this. The Chinese use them both inside and outside for feng shui purposes. Some schools teach that it is only permissible to place the Pa Kua mirror outside the living area. In other places, these mirrors are sometimes hung up within the rooms in droves.

There are four schools in feng shui: the Compass School, the 8 House Method, the School of the Flying Star (Ki), and the Color/Form School. Each of theses four branches of feng shui is established. The longer a person is involved with feng shui, the more the individual schools begin to merge with each other. We can imagine that each of the four feng shui directions is a bowl with a colored elixir of knowledge. If we pour all four elixirs together, then the color dissolves and everything becomes clear, translucent, and transparent. However, those who cling to one extreme will never be able to find the pure water since the teaching of feng shui contains all the important values like tolerance, respect, and inner greatness.

The foundation for every decision is knowledge about the effect of the remedy. Only those who have comprehended how something functions can make their individual decisions about whether they would like to employ the respective accessories.

There are a few simple explanations for the differing statements about feng shui remedies that can already clear up a large portion of the confusion:

Hearsay

A remedy always serves to optimize and improve a living situation. The more specific the remedy is, the more specific its effect on the living situation will be. If I decide to place a mirror at an angle on the wall so it can brighten a dead corner in the room with its captured sunbeams, this certainly doesn't mean it is advisable for everyone else to hang up a mirror at an angle. However, if the owner of an optimized room talks about his success with the crooked mirror in his euphoria, it won't take long until at least 10 people imitate this mirror story. And like a snowball turns into an avalanche, this "secret tip" is spread around until it finally becomes standard advice. However, the knowledge about the application of the mirror is lacking. Unfortunately, in some places the good energy will immediately be returned to the outside world and the effect is everything but positive. Everyone has long forgotten the original living situation where the use of the crooked mirror was meaningful.

The Big Country of China

One further reason for the various kinds of advice can be found in the geography of China. China is larger than the United States of America and all of Europe. The life situations in the east, west, south, and north are not even slightly comparable. It is therefore also not astonishing that completely different things possess a central and vital status in the north than in the south. Once you have learned a bit more about the remedies, you will also be capable of classifying even these pieces of geographical advice more easily. The best way to do this is to imagine the example of a heater. No one would build a house without heating in Germany, but even as far north as Morocco, people are no longer concerned about the cold.

Yet, the theory of feng shui is practiced not only in China and Hong Kong. Another large influence comes from the Land of the Rising Sun. Japanese gardens are probably the most famous ambassadors and show how feng shui can fascinate us outside of closed rooms.

The Fast West

However, I think the main reason that the great variety of remedies has such different messages attached to them is the merging of Eastern culture with Western culture. Within the time span of a few years, we are attempting to translate something into reality that has taken over 4000 years to mature in China. Feng shui articles are copied, produced, and distributed without anyone giving thought to the actual purpose of these things. Some objects look exactly like the Asian prototype but are made from the wrong materials or the central lettering is simply omitted.

A person who builds a house must first focus on the foundation; otherwise, the place will collapse sooner or later. This also applies to us here in the West. Especially in the case of balancing tools with which we would like to optimize our living and working spaces, we should pay attention to accuracy, verifyability, and the knowledge of what is otherwise very important to us in our everyday lives.

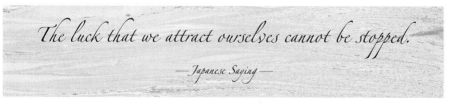

The luck that we attract ourselves cannot be stopped.

— *Japanese Saying* —

Calculating the Zones

There are four different schools of calculation, which we can compare to four different "styles." Most of them work with the *Luo Pan* (feng shui compass) and explain how to divide the home into the nine zones according to the directions. Anyone capable of calculating the sectors with the Luo Pan has enough knowledge to skip this page.

But we would have to add quite a large chapter, the contents and scope of which would go far beyond the limitations of this book*, for those who feel somewhat uncertain about working out the sectors and for those who are completely new to feng shui.

In order for you to find the Relationship Zone in your home or the area of wealth (as well as all of the other zones), the instructions have been simplified as far as possible in the chart below.

Wealth	Fame/ Honor	Relation- ship
Hierarchy	Health	Joy in Life
Knowledge	Path in Life	Helpful Friends

Base line with entrance door

In feng shui, there is a so-called base line, which is the side of your home's floor plan where the entrance door is located (see drawing). Draw the floor plan of your home and divide it into nine fields of equal size. Each room may extend across several sectors since the walls and the feng shui divisions are never identical. If your apartment or house has two entrances, use the one that you consider to be the actual entrance.

If your home does not have a rectangular floor plan, you will recognize that one or more zones are missing. These can be recaptured to a certain degree with the remedies.

You can also consider each individual room from the perspective of its entrance door.

EXAMPLE: When Zone 6 of your apartment is located in a public stairwell or attached to the neighbor's apartment, you can activate the walls that point in the direction of the missing zone with the appropriate balancing tools. In addition, you can take care to powerfully strengthen the area "below—right" in each individual room with the suitable objects. Although this does not give the zone back to you, it does reactivate the supportive energy of the Helpful Friends.

* Further information can be found in: Gerstung and Mehlhase *The Complete Feng Shui Health Handbook*, Lotus Press · Shangri-La 2000

The Three Sources of Power

Even the largest river has its source in a small and powerful spring.
In our homes there are also three sources of good energy.
How we deal with these three sources and thereby stimulate the flow of
chi energy in our rooms is totally up to us.

Fresh Air

Air provides us with oxygen so that we can
live in the first place. If there is too little
oxygen in a room, we experience the air as
sticky, musty, and stale. In workrooms,
the potential for performance sinks to an
absolute low and we immediately feel the
desire to air the room. However, not only
the lack of oxygen prompts us to reach toward the window to open it but also bad
smells. In every home, in addition to the
bathroom, the neuralgic point is also the
kitchen since the cooking smells infiltrate
the other rooms. Smokers put an abrupt
end to fresh air, and some hobby rooms in
which people solder, paint, varnish, and

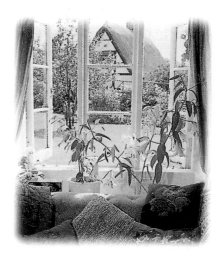

glue are enveloped in acrid air. Human scents can also weaken the air. Our
natural body odors (sweat) are the primary factors here, followed by occasional
vapors that are usually triggered by what we eat. Diseases also have their own
smells and cause the air to become heavy and stagnant.

There are also many causes for the air losing its freshness. In any case, airing
on a regular basis is the simplest solution. However, certain rooms need extra
help. Some bathrooms must constantly stockpile an entire family's dirty laundry.
In addition to personal hygiene and changing the clothes worn directly on the
body (including socks, stockings, and t-shirts) every day, essential oils dripped
onto fragrance stones are a major remedy in bathrooms. In the kitchen, the main
source of relief is the stove ventilator; however, nothing can be drawn away during
cooking if there isn't one in the kitchen. Many people spontaneously open the
window, and this is a very practical solution. Yet, even after meals when the dishes
have been washed, a central "scent cleansing" is necessary since the pots and pans
in particular will otherwise still smell like used oils and fats hours later. The

garbage can should not be forgotten since much of what we throw away has "smelly" qualities. The higher the temperatures are outside, the more frequently the garbage bag should be changed.

In sick-rooms, it is helpful to use essential oils and change the patient's clothing on a regular basis.

Warmth

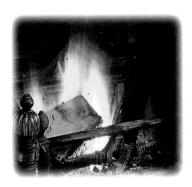

There are recommended values for room temperatures and these range between 73 and 76 degrees F. However, each of us has a very personal temperature sensor that decides whether we feel comfortable or not. This is our sense of warmth. Many people feel absolutely unwell when the temperature is 73 degrees F. They shiver and desperately look for a blanket in which they can snuggle up. In turn, others break out in heat flashes when the temperature hits the 77 degree F mark and walk through their homes barefooted in t-shirts. Even though the differences may be very slight, the various reactions can be quite extreme. During the period in which we heat our homes, we can usually have some input as to how warm we would like to have it.

Temperatures slightly cooler than in the living areas are ideal for healthy sleep, but there shouldn't be a fresh breeze hitting you in the face when you enter the bedroom. Then the result would be not wanting to go to bed out of fear of the cold. A pleasant and cozy warmth is necessary in the living room, where you would like to relax. If it is too cool, then the muscles will cramp and you will be anything but relaxed. It can be slightly cooler in workrooms, but the activities that occur in them are the deciding factor. People who continuously move around and are physically active will get warm while they work. But a person sitting in front of the computer won't be productive if his or her fingers seem to be frozen to the keyboard.

In every household where there are a number of people, different sensitivities to temperature may clash with each other. If all of the family members have almost the same wavelength, this is naturally the perfect situation. But if there are different sensitivities, the temperature may have a disruptive effect on the sense of well-being. If there is enough space available and each member of the family has his or her own room, then each can be the master of the heater in his or her own domain. Then it is sensible to find a compromised level of warmth acceptable to all the family members in the living room and other mutual living areas.

Even today, the most wonderful source of heat is the visible fire. The location of a tiled stove, a Swedish oven, or a fireplace should be as central as possible so that the warmth of the fire can radiate in all directions like a shining sun. Even if open fireplaces now fulfill more of an elegant decorative than an elemental purpose in many modern apartments and houses because the rooms are centrally heated, it is still important to use then on a regular basis during the cold seasons. An oven that does not burn is a symbol of "extinguished" fire.

Light

There are three main sources of energy that allow the good chi to blossom in our living areas and workrooms. Light (in addition to warmth and fresh air) is probably the most interesting because most of us have enormous potential that can be optimized in a wonderful way.

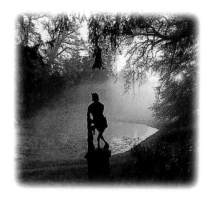

We are usually not accustomed to experimenting with light and not particularly familiar with the play of light and shadow (shadow play—silhouettes). Shadow-play theater, as performed in Bali, Indonesia, and many other Asiatic countries, is difficult to find in Western nations.

Even silhouettes, which create a fascination through fullness and emptiness (or also light and shadow) only accompany us into the lower grades at school. As a result, we have never developed a culture for this art and it is difficult for us to create silhouettes with paper and scissors.

Consequently, it isn't surprising that our living areas do not integrate this interplay and we find the same forms of illumination over and over again:

The hallway usually has a plain ceiling lamp with a simple design, sometimes acquired from the previous occupant. The light it provides is usually less than spectacular. Standard lamps are generally found in the living rooms, usually standing next to the sofa and illuminating the ceiling in accordance with the brightness of the dimmer setting. We often find the classic hanging lamps above the dining-room table and in other rooms. These may have an outdated form or prove to be less than high quality in their structure. This may all sound a bit mean and cynical, but is a common situation. Finding a suitable lamp usually means an extended search. The ones we like the most are frequently too expensive, yet they will accompany us through many years.

Since light plays a major role in feng shui, here are a few tips:

Light in the Kitchen

We prepare our food in the kitchen and the amount of light there determines how well we can see what we do. However, the quality of the light can also contribute a great deal toward how we experience the food and how we ultimately treat it. Whether fruit, meat, or vegetables, our food will smile at us and be appealing depends upon the lighting. Then we enjoy being in the kitchen, create a positive eating culture, and therefore make a valuable contribution to our health. This increases our sense of well-being. In the negative situation, the meals are unappetizing, we cook less, and then eat quickly and without much enjoyment.

Light in the Bathroom

If you have ever had to use the bathroom at a train station, you will probably not have a pleasant memory of the toilet there. However, this is not necessarily a hygiene issue but mainly related to the bluish-cold lighting that causes us to keep our visit as short as possible. However, if we have ever had the opportunity to use the restroom in a luxury hotel, we will have a positive memory of the golden light with golden tones of the mirror there. Although we may not see things as clearly in that mirror, the light flatters our skin and surrounds us with a shimmer of warmth and a touch of elegance. The situation in our homes is very similar and our choice of light can determine how much we enjoy our visit to the bathroom. If the washstand cabinet has neon lighting, it is best to immediately replace the cold-light tube with a warm-light tube.

Light in the Corridor

In some apartment floor plans, the hallway runs through the middle of the apartment and subdivides the remaining areas into different rooms. Hall lighting fixtures are usually sad creations without any illuminating power or esthetics. However, once we become aware that the center of any home corresponds to health, then the hall lighting quickly becomes a central theme. The lamp in the middle of the home has the function of a sun that wants to send its power into all of the adjoining rooms. The more radiant the sun, the greater its energy will be.

Light in the Living Areas

You must experience a sense of well-being in the living areas. This is the primary basic rule. The light must correspond with the needs that you want to live to the full in each respective room: quality lighting for watching TV, good and bright light for reading, and warm light for cuddling. However, the light should not be blinding. If you like spots or little halogen lamps, be sure to direct them so that no one is "blinded" when looking at them. Hanging lamps with bulbs that are not covered by lamp shades can also be changed and refined through the proper choice of a bulb.

Dead Corners

Every home has a "dead corner" somewhere. These are areas in which, among other things, dust likes to collect. The energy cannot circulate freely in a corner and this area usually becomes limp and the walls darken in the course of time. A standard lamp will cover such corners very well, but salt-crystal lamps are also the ideal helpers for dead corners. With a bit of aptitude, a few plants, and one of these lamps, a limp corner can become a comfortable retreat.

Valuable Treasures, Pictures, and Decorative Objects

We human beings are all gatherers and hunters, so each of us has carried some treasures and decorative objects into our homes during the course of time. Quite frequently, these dear things simply gather dust and their auras become weaker and weaker. Light and treasures are ideal partners. Whether you explicitly light up a figurine from the ceiling or create an empty space in a bookcase for a decorative object (and thereby loosen up a massive wall) and additionally illuminate the object, you are activating the energy of joy in any case. There are special curved lamps to install above the frames of pictures. Some rooms are completely changed just by illuminating the pictures on the wall.

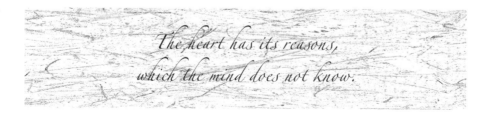

The heart has its reasons,
which the mind does not know.

Symbols of Love
Balsam for Heart and Soul

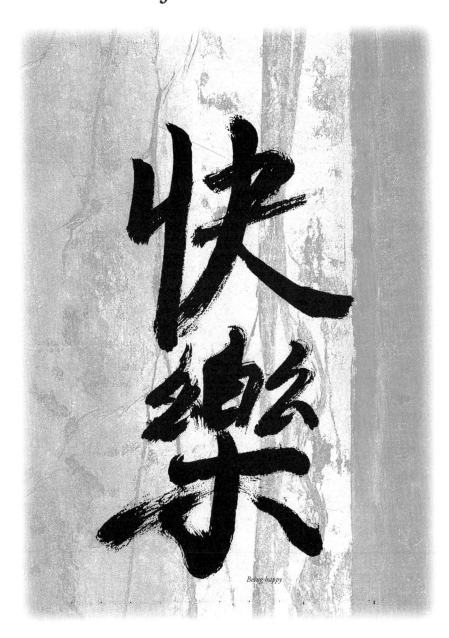

Being happy

Love is the greatest source of our vital energy. It provides us with happiness, joy, contentment, strength, and warmth. Yet, the wellspring of love does not bubble constantly and in a consistent flow. Sometimes it almost completely stops its activities for a certain period of time.

When a relationship seems to become boring, tired, and weak, acquaintances only last a short amount of time, or the vital spark does not catch fire, you can approach these situations with the supportive power of the love symbols.

In feng shui, Zone 2 is the area of relationship and love. But these feelings also appear in Zone 7 (Joy in Life), 4 (Inner Wealth), and 3 (Family).

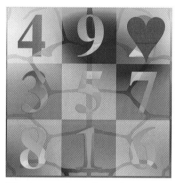

The Relationship Zone is found at the "back right," which applies to both the entire home and the individual rooms.

Before you begin placing the symbols of love as supportive power in Zone 2, it is important to first check what is already located there. When I am invited to consultations, the theme of love is very often the reason for my visit. On the basis of the following examples, I would like to show you how we portray feelings in a "hidden" manner, which then oppress our hearts.

The entrance door is located on this line.

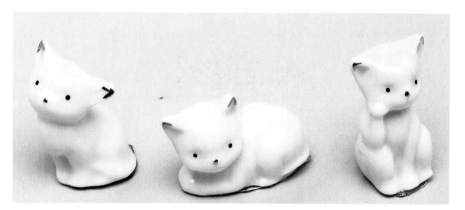

The three porcelain figures all look in a different direction, as if they had nothing to say to each other. Only the smallest of the three figures attempts to create a connection. The client's family consisted of two adults and a pet. The little cat was actually the connecting link between the two people, who had emotionally turned away from each other.

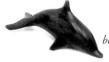

The two dolphins cannot find the way to each other because an insurmountable obstacle stands between them.

19

Pair of Dolphins

The eagle, the bear, and the dolphin have one thing in common: they live, they exist, and they are actually very normal animals. And yet, they are much, much more. While the unicorn and the dragon connect us with other spheres, the dolphin has become a close friend here on earth. Even ancient legends and sagas tell of the dolphins' cleverness as they show humanity the path to enlightenment and accompany us on it.

The loving and caring way in which dolphins treat each other and the same type of open and cheerful encounter with us humans is an ideal feng shui symbol for the entire area of partnership. Pictures, wind chimes, window pictures, figurines, and the individual arrangement in which two or even more dolphins are found, help support us in finding the path to ourselves, to other people, friends, relatives, colleagues at work, as well as agencies and authorities in a loving, open, and harmonious manner.

The most ideal location is Zone 2 (Relationship), but all of the other zones can also be activated by a pair of dolphins. More joy in the relationship: Zone 7; more wealth in love: Zone 4; inner strength through the partnership: Zone 5; a strong (winning) team: Zones 9 + 1; learning from each other (Knowledge): Zone 8; being there for each other (Friends): Zone 6; being inseparably connected (Hierarchy): Zone 3.

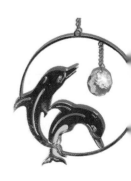

Dolphins are also symbols of the strength, the joy, and the serenity from the element of water, which represents communication and understanding, among other things.

Wedding Photo

The wedding photo is a remembrance of a day that is certain to be absolutely extraordinary. All photos, even those with a less spectacular background (mutual vacation, etc.) are great providers of good energy since they remind us of specific moments and special feelings in our life. Even those who are not married to their partner are certain to particularly love a photo with a similar ideal value. Partnership photos are great chi providers, but only as long as they can radiate. If the pictures and frames are dusty, the chi will disappear as well.

If you are not inclined to cleaning, then it is better to make a photo album to place on a shelf in the Relationship Zone. As an honest confession of weakness in the area of housekeeping, this decision has nothing in common with the negative statement of "wanting to lock away the relationship" and is therefore absolutely sound and legitimate.

Candles

The fire of love can be depicted in no better way than by two burning candles in Zone 2 (Relationship).

If your heart's desire for a relationship has remained unfulfilled, you can place two candles in one open bowl. This symbolizes your openness for love. The ideal color of the bowl is either green or lilac, even thought this may not appear to be particularly elegant. A more attractive approach is to select either a glass bowl or a black container (element of water) and place fresh green leaves (element of wood = growing and thriving) in with the candles.

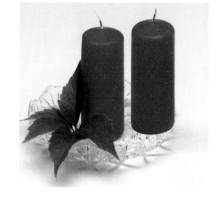

One very important factor is the structure of the candles that are lit for love. If the candles flicker, hiss, and produce a long flame, this portrays a fiery, hot relationship. Candles that burn slowly symbolize that long and steady, but less fiery path of togetherness and relationship.

Even the form and the color have an additional, deeper significance. This example should show you that a simple starting position in feng shui can quickly become a very complex matter in which every detail is important.

However, there is another basis for decision-making: When selecting the candles, act intuitively "from your gut." There are no coincidences, or, in other words: What you would like to express will also "occur" to you.

The Dragon and the Phoenix

When a dragon and a phoenix are portrayed together, they no longer represent just the elements of wood and fire but are a symbol for man and woman. In heaven, they have entered into a union for life and are connected for all of eternity. This heavenly and eternal bond is found in numerous Chinese illustrations and on Chinese decorations. The ideal places for them are in Zone 2 (Relationship), as well as the bedroom. (Only the dragon is pictured here.)

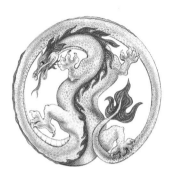

Doves

We say that two people in love are acting "lovey-dovey," and doves are a symbol for peace (a white dove) throughout the entire world. Two doves represent faithfulness, longevity, and love. The more they move in the same direction together or the closer they are together, the stronger their connection will be. However, they should never fly away from each other or show each other a "cold shoulder" if they are meant to be a symbol of love. All animal pictures, no matter whether two turtledoves, two elephants, or two cats are depicted, have an especially lovely effect in the Relationship Zone and naturally also in the bedroom. In any other living area, they intensify the togetherness and the unity of the relationship.

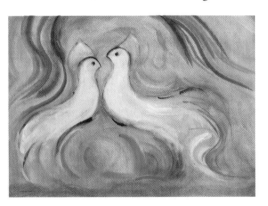

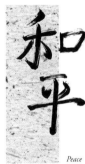

Peace

Two Rings

Just as in the West, rings are a double symbol of love in China as well. In the Partnership Zone, calligraphy depicting two circles also symbolizes unending, eternal love.

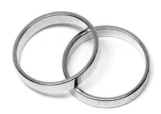

The following symbols, which have detailed significance for love and partnership, can upgrade various zones:

Good-Luck Coins	Crystal-Glass Spirals	Yin Yang
A good-luck coin is a talisman of luck and contains: love, peace, health, and money. If you would specifically like to activate love, you can waken the energy of the heart and the feelings with this talisman of luck. The good-luck coin is often hung in the window of the Relationship Zone. See page 39 for more details about the good-luck coin.	The two coils of the crystal-glass spirals additionally symbolize the power of duality in the Relationship Zone. Just like the endless knot or the infinity sign, the crystal-glass spiral in the partnership area is representative of eternal love and the related relationship that is inseparable at all times. See pages 73-75 for more about spirals.	Wherever balance and harmony are desired, the Yin Yang supports this message. In Zone 2, the Yin Yang represents a balanced relationship and a harmonious distribution of the forces between the partners. Responsibility, trust, love and respect, tolerance and generosity—everything in a harmonious balance. See page 79 for more about Yin Yang.

The Supportive Path to Money and Wealth

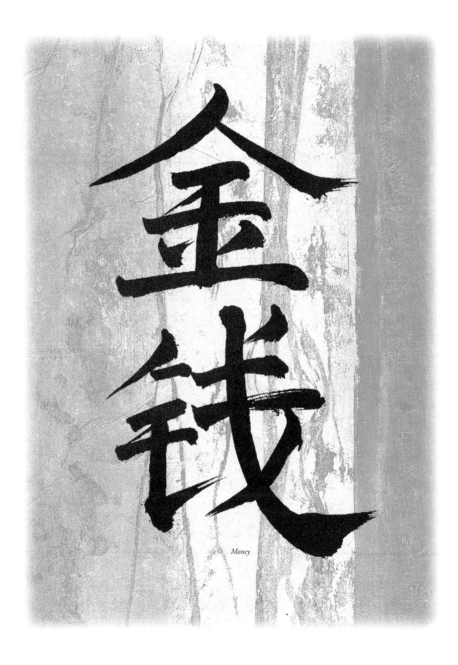

Money

A certain amount of money, wealth, and material goods are essential for all of us so that we can regulate our obligations like rent, insurance, and other costs and can acquire the vital necessities like food and clothing. Everything that remains after that is at our disposal and we can let ourselves be seduced by the things that we like, that we enjoy, and that we simply want to have.

However, we are all naturally tempted by many expensive or luxurious things that not only place a considerable strain on our budget but would perhaps also wipe it out. It is therefore not surprising that activating the Wealth Zone in particular has a long tradition behind it.

An extravagant vacation, a great car, beautiful furniture—all of this is not absolutely necessary, but it does enrich our lives. This enrichment is not only material but also in our hearts because we enjoy it. In feng shui, money and wealth represent not only the external, purely material aspect, but also inner wealth and our contentment.

Zone 4 is the area of inner and outer wealth in feng shui.

Since the forces of the Wealth Zone are not only related to the material energies and money, it is absolutely necessary to first check the current state of this area. Perhaps you have picked up something that you would like to dispense with. An "undesired wealth" has manifested itself here in various consultations.

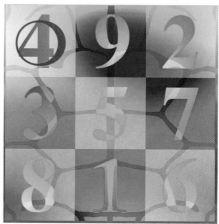

The Wealth Zone is found at the "back left," which applies to both the entire home and for each individual room.

The entrance door is on this line

Aquariums

If you walk through the streets of Hong Kong or visit an Asian enterprise in the West, you will quickly discover that there is an aquarium in almost every business. This applies whether it is a car dealer, a restaurant, or a clothing store. Aquariums are probably the most intensive example for the perfect mixture of feng shui and superstition. In the colloquial Chinese, there is an expression for money that sounds almost like the word for "flowing away." If water cannot flow away, as in

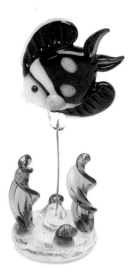

an aquarium where the water is collected as a symbol for money, this is advantageous for its owner. The brighter, larger, and healthier the fish are, the more colorful, splendid, and longer the person's life will be. Ideally, eight fish swim in the water. Seven of these are colorful and the eighth fish is black because "it eats up what is evil." Since aquariums are usually also illuminated, the white gravel glitters and the plants and decorations create a beautiful ambiance. This creates a perfect dream world, a type of paradise on earth, within a very small space.

The Money Tree

In May, many people tie loops and ribbons onto the trees, which looks wonderful. These colorful ribbons are used through the year in feng shui in order to activate the elements and zones. The most familiar of these is probably the money tree. A little boxtree (buxus) is used with its trunk and the bush is cut into a small sphere. The trunk symbolizes growth, the sphere is the world in harmony, and the round form represents the coins. This then expresses a harmonious growth of the forces. A white ribbon attached to the upper part of the trunk, right beneath the bush, stands for repeating the element of metal (round form) and for the desired money.

Just as the ribbons play in the wind, the energy of the money is awakened to life in a playful way.

It is best to also include little decorations in the colors of the elements fire (red/orange), earth (yellow), and water (blue/black) in the pot so that the creative cycle of the elements can be completed again.

The ideal location for the money tree is Zone 4, which symbolizes wealth.

The money tree can naturally also be transformed into its less familiar relatives, the love tree and the power tree. The love tree always has two birds, sitting together in a very tender way, on wires added to the tree. The ribbons are not white here, but a delicate pink (gentle growth) and red (the fire of love). The power tree strengths any zone in which it is placed. The ribbons are either multicolored, so that all of the elements are represented, or totally green. Instead of a "pair of lovers," strong power symbols like the sun, small crystals, or the Yin Yang are attached to the tree. The form of the sphere (universe) is also used for both of these variations.

26

The Glass Bowl

Many people throw their change into bowls in the evening or collect larger amounts of it in glass vases for their vacations. Then, depending on its location, the following happens: The containers become full or they are forgotten. Or they are constantly plundered. What we simply do as a "game," has become a mature method in feng shui for activating the attraction, the intensity, and the flow of money energy. Anyone who wants to amass wealth should not place the bowl in a location where nothing happens or where something will be constantly removed from it. The ideal location is Zone 4, which (just like the Relationship Zone and all the other zones) can also be activated in each individual room, if necessary.

A basic rule in feng shui is to never use a vase with a narrow neck to collect the money energy. The narrower the door through which the wealth is intended to flow, the less can enter it. An open bowl is therefore ideal. The material of the bowl also plays a large role. A metal container is clearly focused on money, while a glass bowl or a black bowl transforms the energy by an additional step, into the abundance of inner and outer wealth. However, the main point is the content of the bowl. It is absolutely senseless to place very small coins in it. A person who activates small forces will only harvest small amounts of money. If you place postage stamps into the bowl, you will also receive large quantities of mail but perhaps also the type that you don't even want. So the first step is to consider what you experience as wealth in a very personal way. Objects that represent inner wealth are naturally also suitable for the bowl.

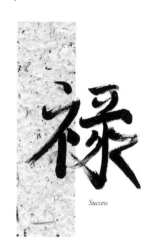

Success

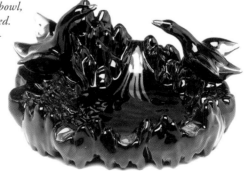

Place a few folded currency bills in this black bowl, so that the total amount can be clearly recognized. The sum of money, presented in this way, symbolizes that the person is in good financial shape. Both of the ducks (ducks have lifelong partnerships) represent the wealth of love and feelings.

However, in classical feng shui, only money and material values are found in these bowls. Unfortunately, inner wealth and contentment are sometimes nearly "forgotten" in all of the striving for money.

Pile of Gold Coins

The pile of gold coins is one of my favorite symbols with respect to the flow of money. The five coins are attached to each other in a little pile and the upper two have a clear and appealing Chinese inscription on them. Translated literally, the proverb on the coins says: "May wealth flow to you from all sides." However, in colloquial language, the translation is warmly and pleasantly transformed into the following saying:

May the coins jump into your pocket.

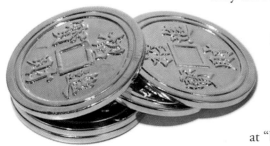

The pile of gold coins is a symbol, which is primarily at home in Zone 4 and mainly addresses material wealth. At every workplace where economic interests are in the foreground (or should not be forgotten), this pile of coins on the desk is an excellent support. When you sit at the desk, the location for it is at "back left," in Zone 4 of the desk surface.

Water

Clean, clear, and flowing water or fountains that have water of drinking quality are not only the equivalent of something valuable in feng shui. In the entire world, water has an outstandingly high value. Without water, neither plants nor flowers thrive; human beings and animals also die of thirst without it. Most people in Western nations are very fortunate to turn on the tap and have drinking water flow out of it as long as they like. However, we should not forget that when the teaching of feng shui developed—and even into the 21st century—the situation was completely different. Even today, not all the residents of Hong Kong have running water (the Aberdeen Boat People). It also isn't surprising that water and wealth (money) are equated with each other.

A room fountain is therefore more than just an elegant way of keeping their room air moist. According to feng shui, it is also an extreme luxury item since it bears the source of life within itself. Consequently, great care should always be given to always maintaining these fountains.

In order to further increase good fortune, coins that are thrown into the fountain can awaken wishes to life. If a fountain is located in the Relationship Zone, the source of life will be connected with love; in the Wealth Zone, the material level is activated and inner forces are strengthened in the area of health.

You can activate and strengthen every zone with the symbol of water that is moving (but not flowing away). However, if you have the feeling that money is flowing through your fingers, that the relationship is "watery," or you are "drifting" in a situation in your life, then the existing water represents too much of a good thing. In these situations, it is recommended that you work with stable and steady remedies. The element of earth is excellently suited as a good foundation here.

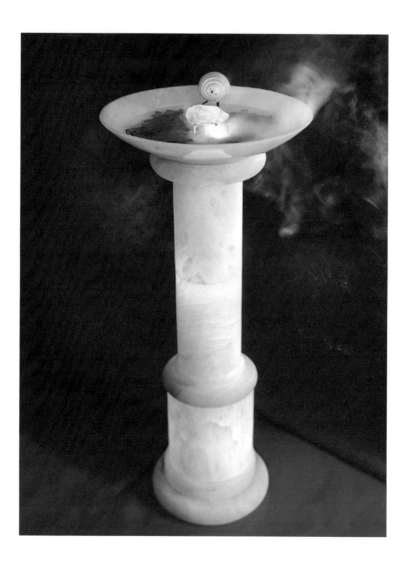

Various symbols can be used in an all-purpose manner. According to where they are placed, they achieve a deeper meaning. Here is a detailed explanation on the specific topics of money and wealth:

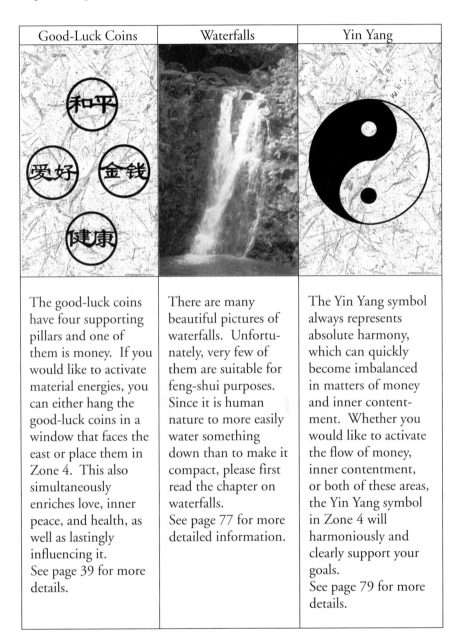

Good-Luck Coins	Waterfalls	Yin Yang
The good-luck coins have four supporting pillars and one of them is money. If you would like to activate material energies, you can either hang the good-luck coins in a window that faces the east or place them in Zone 4. This also simultaneously enriches love, inner peace, and health, as well as lastingly influencing it. See page 39 for more details.	There are many beautiful pictures of waterfalls. Unfortunately, very few of them are suitable for feng-shui purposes. Since it is human nature to more easily water something down than to make it compact, please first read the chapter on waterfalls. See page 77 for more detailed information.	The Yin Yang symbol always represents absolute harmony, which can quickly become imbalanced in matters of money and inner contentment. Whether you would like to activate the flow of money, inner contentment, or both of these areas, the Yin Yang symbol in Zone 4 will harmoniously and clearly support your goals. See page 79 for more details.

Protection and Power for the House and Its People

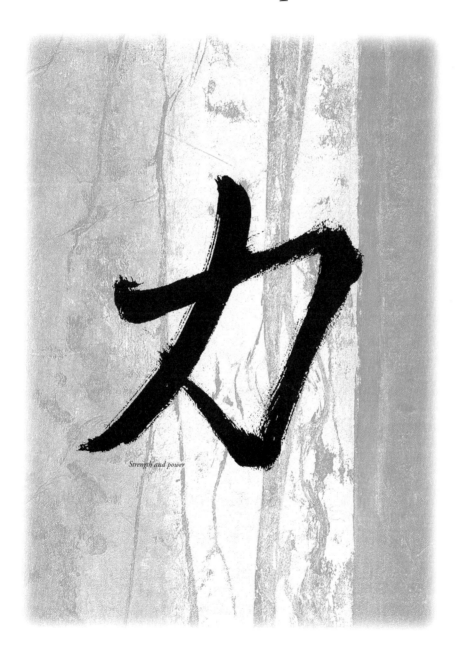

Strength and power

Protectors and Guardians

Protectors and bodyguards are not just for human beings. For hundreds of years, houses and important buildings in Asia have also had their protectors. However, these are not made of flesh and blood but stone. They have fear-inspiring faces and muscular bodies. They are called Foo and are a mixture of a lion and a dragon. In the West, we mainly see them at Chinese restaurants. They always

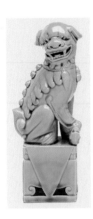

appear as a pair of twins and are posed to the right and left of the entrance door. It is their task to probe the mind and intentions of the entering guest for purity. It is said that people with good thoughts can pass by the Foos unhindered, but they see through bad people and refuse them entry.

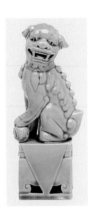

So if you wish to enter a house that has the Foo brothers in front of it, first consciously examine the purity of your thoughts in order to enter the building in peace and with a noble heart.

Rose Globes

Rose globes protect the occupant of a house from negative energies that emanate from the neighbors or uninvited guests or are transmitted to the property through the traffic on the road. Rose globes have the same type of energetic effect as the convex Pa Kua mirrors. Imagine placing a bowl upside down in the sink and then turning on the tap. The water runs down the outside of the bowl, is diverted away from it, and its flow is therefore weakened. If you turn on the tap even further so that a powerful stream of water comes out, the water will even spray away from the bowl. And this is exactly what happens with negative energies. Energies that are only slightly negative will be diverted, but strongly negative energies will bounce off and be diffused in all directions.

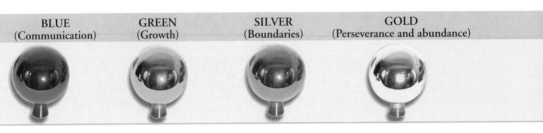

| BLUE (Communication) | GREEN (Growth) | SILVER (Boundaries) | GOLD (Perseverance and abundance) |

However, not only the form of the rose globe has a protective effect. The size and color allow its message to become even more precise, concrete, and purposeful:

Here are a few examples: If your neighbors are very curious, then it's best to use a *silver* globe in order to achieve a clear boundary. In the vicinity of churches (confession of sins, penance, and evil deeds), as well as hospitals (illness, suffering, and death), you can counteract the heavy thoughts of the visitors with the color *mint* or protect your own joy in life with *orange*. You can naturally also achieve a boundary with the color silver. If your relationship to neighbors tends to be somewhat reserved, then *green* and *blue* will help in any case.

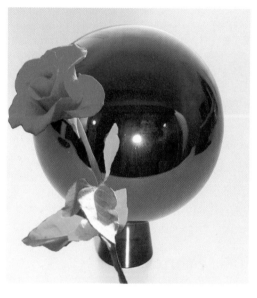

If negative energy is directed toward you through a street, then your are primarily at the mercy of the traffic. Of course, there are also possible solutions for this situation. However, never place a red globe directly in front of the entrance to your home. If you do this, it will signal a very dangerous message to drivers—namely, that reaching your entrance is a major goal for them. The best color to use in this case is again silver in order to set clear boundaries. You can use red if these globes are placed at the outer edges of the property. With it you produce steam (fire and water) in the circle of elements, which confuses the drivers and causes them to drive more slowly. There is good reason for always using a combination of the colors red and white for the street signs related to danger.

However, you can not only guide negative energies away from your home with the rose globes, but your own needs and desires may also simply flow away. If a room has too many windows, a large amount of energy will also be lost. A rose globe in the flowerpot guides the energy that would normally flow out through the window back into the room, which keeps it in the room. The choice of the

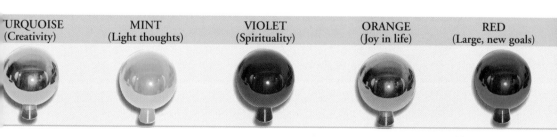

URQUOISE (Creativity)	MINT (Light thoughts)	VIOLET (Spirituality)	ORANGE (Joy in life)	RED (Large, new goals)

color is of greatest significance, and this should not be considered a permanent situation. So don't regret replacing the current color that is no longer appropriate with a new, more suitable one when you have new goals, new desires, and new priorities.

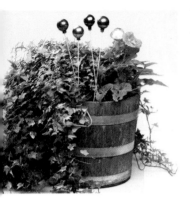

Here are a few examples: When you have the feeling that you could do more with your life, then you have the choice of three colors that could be helpful to you: green for continuous, rather slow but constant inner and also outer (professional) growth, mint for new ideas and creative impetus, and violet (eggplant) for inner, spiritual, and mental development. If you have accepted the challenge of further education, a new job, a career opportunity, or even the path of self-employment, then the color red will help you to achieve the goals and the color orange will help you to not lose your courage and joy in life despite the great burden. Artistic talents are best supported by mint and violet. If you would like to support the expressive power of your voice and speech, then use the color blue. Discussion groups also benefit from blue and violet. There is power in peacefulness, and the color gold is ideal for stabilizing inner and outer wealth. It furnishes strength, self-confidence, and self-assurance. Moreover, the color gold helps people achieve an aura of dignity, which can be invaluable to those who are at the mercy of other people's moods.

Stones

Stones have a very important meaning in Asia and in feng shui. There are often large stones with proverbs written on them in the mountains, at the edges of streets, at the entrance to towns, and at bridges. The text is always related to a story. An emperor once had the word "loyalty" written on a stone near his city in order to eternally emphasize the connection to his country.

However, not only towns and landscapes with stones that have written texts are given an abiding place in the culture of China. Houses are also protected and guarded by a very special stone. You cannot purchase this special stone that protects and strengthens the house, the property, and its occupants.

If your house is not guarded by an imposing stone, then you can search for one. Very special stones detach themselves from their subsoil time and again in forests, near rivers, and in the mountains—and would like to be taken home by a person who knows how to appreciate their powers. A protective stone is always 6 inches or larger and its form usually corresponds with the element of the person to be protected. A spontaneous love and connection occurs between the person and the stone. When you stand in front of the appropriate relic, then you will recognize it. Even if it may be difficult to carry it home or put it into your car: For the one hour of effort, dragging it home, and muscle aches, the stone will protect you for a lifetime!

Many old pieces of property have a stone that someone once placed there many generations ago. In this case, the house has already found its protective stone. In no case should you remove this old guardian, even if you prefer to have arranged something more modern. If you have no choice than to move the protective stone, be sure to select a place for it that has a higher quality and more beautiful appearance than its current location.

Signboards

Wooden signboards are a widespread remedy for protecting houses since it is much easier to paint letters on them with a brush than chisel them into a stone. Just like engravings in stone, the texts sometimes have a rather strange content since people

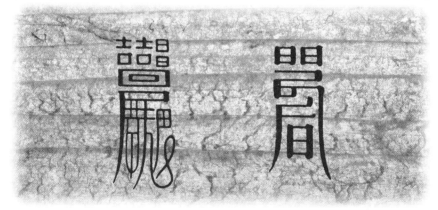

also like to use an individual sentence out of an entire story as the core statement on wooden signboards.

However, not only "encoded messages" are written on the signboards, but also magical signs and direct statements.

Here is a small selection of the most famous signs. You can also draw them on the wooden signboards with a brush—it's not very difficult to do. The best size for the little board is about 12 inches high and about 4 inches wide. If necessary, you can change the dimensions to adapt to the Chinese character, which is a common practice. Above all, it is important that it have a flawless appearance when it is done.

Special Symbols of Good Fortune

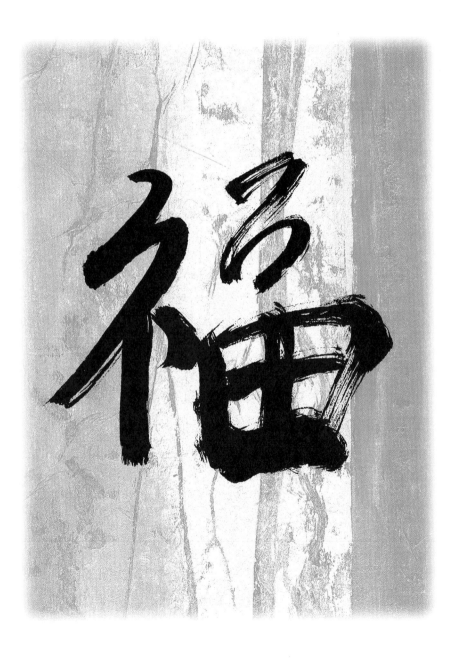

Good-Luck Bags

Little red bags, which are embroidered in exquisite gold decoration, are given as presents on numerous occasions in Asia. These little red bags are put to use at weddings, birthdays, and other important events. Depending on the occasion, there are normally smaller or larger currency bills in them.

These good-luck bags are also employed in feng shui. The consultant naturally does not give his clients money but puts a saying that is very valuable for the occupant in this wrapper. In many areas of China, it is even a custom for people to leave the good-luck bags that the feng shui masters have given to them sealed or closed, in the same state as they were received. The closed little bag is then hung up or lovingly placed at a central spot in the home. The luck that has been packed into this little bag by the feng shui master should not escape, so it is held for an entire lifetime in this way.

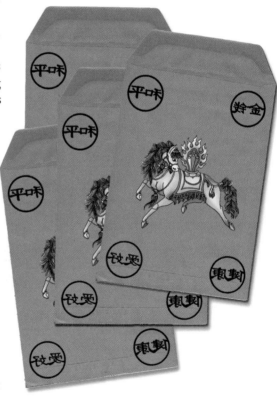

In the West, the good-luck bags have been used very sparingly by feng shui consultants since these little bags are still something of a "secret tip." Whatever is in this packaging of bright China red and gold, everyone (even in the West) is happy to receive them. Children, whether in China or elsewhere, love to receive these little bags since they already sense, quite correctly, that something valuable (like a lovely present or even a currency bill) is hidden within it.

Every gift that is packaged in a good-luck bag automatically becomes more valuable and elegant. The special touch of the coloration naturally also contributes to this effect since, even here, nothing is left to "chance."

In China and Hong Kong, good-luck bags are as widespread in every household as paper handkerchiefs are in the West. They usually come in packages of 20, 50, or 100 pieces per set. Anyone who does feng shui professionally or loves special things, will certainly be unable to resist this beautiful Asian custom in the long run.

Ladybugs

In many cultures, beetles have a very special power and qualities attributed to them. These usually seem completely irrational when we attempt to find the secret of the legends. There are neither stories nor sensible reasons why this specific bug should have been seen as the messenger of luck or joy.

Since we rarely see Chinese beetles in the West, the entire story only takes on a meaning for us when we think of our own good-luck beetle: the ladybug. These little bugs with the black heads, the red body, and black dots bring good cheer and good luck to anyone they land on.

Many people who are interested in feng shui are somewhat afraid that their home could look "slightly Chinese" after a consultation. Hanging up lucky dragons, Yin Yang symbols, fans, and flutes and decorating the walls with Far Eastern culture naturally doesn't correspond to everyone's taste.

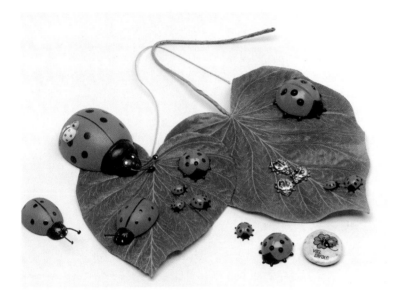

However, we can remain in our own regions since there are excellent good-luck symbols available as alternatives. Horseshoes, which catch good luck like a bowl, have a basic thought behind them that is similar to the good-luck bags, but the statement is not as direct and precise. Our four-leafed clover is another Western symbol.

A very popular symbol in German culture is the clover leaf with a ladybug on it. Together, these two good-luck symbols result in doubled good-luck.

It is always fascinating to see how such different cultures create symbols that are nearly identical in meaning but could hardly be more different in terms of their appearance.

The clover leaf with the ladybug is one of the most frequently used good-luck charms in German-speaking countries. Even if it is very small, it is still a symbol of doubled good luck.

The Good-Luck Coin

The good-luck coin is a talisman of luck—a symbol of the harmonious interplay of peace, love, money, and health.

The union of these four cornerstones form the foundation for a fulfilled life. The inner, as well as the outer, wealth is harmoniously increased and balanced and the path to the intimate other, to our fellow human beings and friends, is filled with love and peace. The earthly home of the soul—our body—is blessed with health so that our desired, goals, and ideas can be realized and fulfilled in this world.

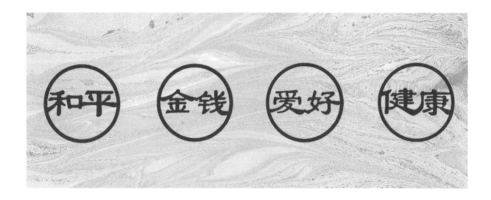

When the sun shines upon the rainbow crystal at the center of the good-luck coin, it appears that the four circles of luck begin to radiate and fill the observer with all their powers.

If the good-luck coins are used according to the teachings of the Chinese harmony theory of feng shui, they can support and promote the goals of the home's occupants in the zones of relationship and wealth. Unfortunately, the center of each home, which is associated with health, often does not enjoy any sunshine because walls prevent it from entering. The good-luck coin is used here like a picture to give the occupant's health supportive help and the strength necessary for everyday life.

The good-luck coin is a precious symbol since it also bears the values of confidence, courage, strength, and hope within it. When you give someone a good-luck coin, you show your deep respect or affection for them since the statement of the coin is noble and pure. If you give yourself a good-luck coin, you fill your own heart with the highest values so that you can shine like a sun yourself. Your home and surrounding world will be delighted by the warming rays that come from within you.

The Classical Remedies and Symbols in Feng Shui

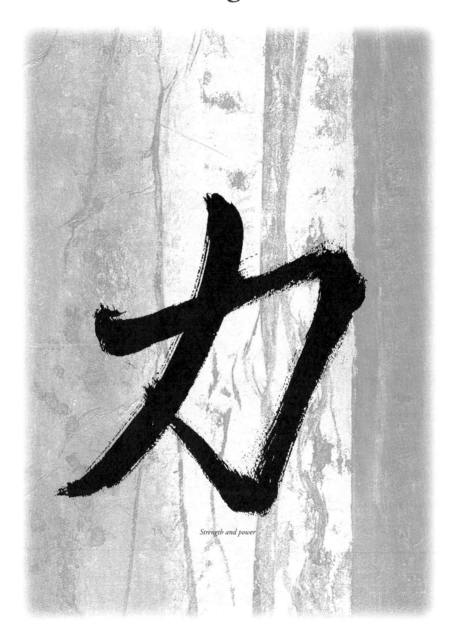

Strength and power

Old Man

The depiction of the old man is always a symbol of longevity. This naturally means spending your old age in prosperity, strong physical and mental health, and without worries. The symbol of longevity is frequently used and is coupled with a rather widely ranging wish list. Fish also mean good luck and wealth, so it isn't surprising that the old man is frequently depicted as a fisherman with a big fish hanging from his fishing pole (not shown in picture here).

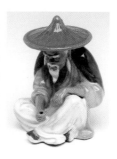

Astrological Signs

We are born in the signs of Virgo, Libra, Sagittarius, or one of the nine other heavenly bodies that change in monthly cycles. The basis of Chinese astrology is the "big year," which lasts for twelve years and contains the twelve earthly branches.

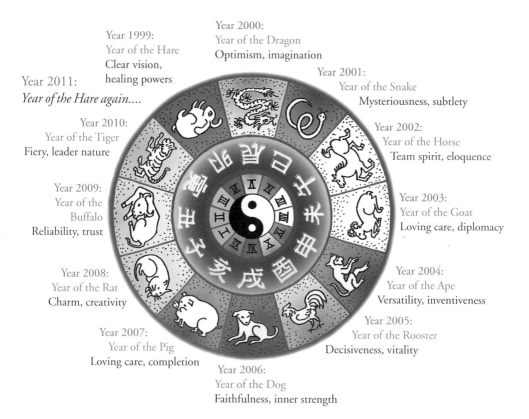

Year 1999:
Year of the Hare
Clear vision,
healing powers

Year 2000:
Year of the Dragon
Optimism, imagination

Year 2011:
Year of the Hare again....

Year 2001:
Year of the Snake
Mysteriousness, subtlety

Year 2010:
Year of the Tiger
Fiery, leader nature

Year 2002:
Year of the Horse
Team spirit, eloquence

Year 2009:
Year of the
Buffalo
Reliability, trust

Year 2003:
Year of the Goat
Loving care, diplomacy

Year 2008:
Year of the Rat
Charm, creativity

Year 2004:
Year of the Ape
Versatility, inventiveness

Year 2007:
Year of the Pig
Loving care, completion

Year 2005:
Year of the Rooster
Decisiveness, vitality

Year 2006:
Year of the Dog
Faithfulness, inner strength

41

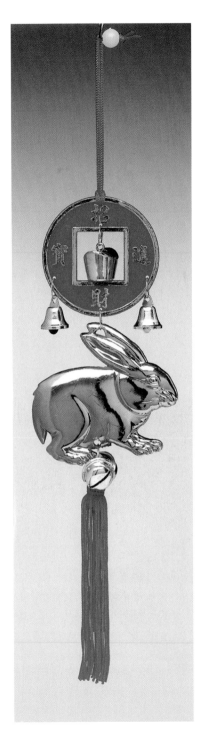

We know these twelve branches as the Chinese Zodiac. (The personal horoscope also contains the four pillars of fate and the inner distribution of the five elements.) Since the entire year stands under the rulership of one of the 12 animals, its nature and character, the new "patron of the year" and its good forces are welcomed in the most hearty manner on the Chinese New Year.

Amulets are hung up on the Chinese New Year in honor of the patron of the year and very frequently remain in place for the entire year until they are replaced by the next animal.

Bamboo

At first glance, bamboo is a very normal plant that grows well and is quite content with little. However, in the Asiatic region, it plays an absolutely paramount role among the thousands of plants that grow and thrive there. Countless works of calligraphy and illustrations are decorated with a picture of bamboo. A quality that we human beings also strive for and seek is ascribed to the bamboo, which explains why it occupies such an unusual and outstanding position:

**If bamboo is bent, it does not break, it yields.
Once we let go of the bamboo, it snaps back and stands as before, upright and proud.**

Softness Subdues the Hard Things in Life

Bamboo is one of the strongest symbols for our path in life. When we are born, we are as supple as bamboo. After our death, we become hard and stiff. During the course of our life, we must also survive some storms and tempests without breaking. Stress, sadness, annoyance, anger, and frustration make us hard and stiff. But the symbol of bamboo represents the strength of being able to let go of this pressure and smoothly follow our path again.

Quite frequently, the bamboo pictures are accompanied by a sun or a moon. Which heavenly body is depicted is not obvious to the observer. In Japan, the sun is still the symbol for the feminine and universal warmth and love. The sun or moon represent our inner voice, our intuitive guidance. There is a wonderful message in the double picture of bamboo/moon and bamboo/sun that tells us we will receive the strength to get back on our feet in life like the bamboo so that we can master all of the difficulties. Furthermore, we never need to feel lonesome because universal love and warmth (sun or moon) accompany us always and eternally.

A calligraphy or window picture with the symbol of bamboo and the crystal as the sun or moon will give us the feeling of confidence and self-assurance on a daily basis. The idea place is the window in the north or the window in the Zone of the Life Path.

Ribbons, Garlands, and Chinese Lamps

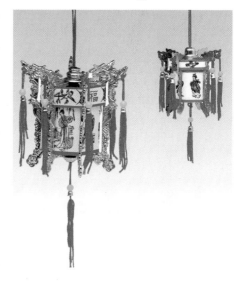

Cheerfully flattering ribbons and little flags, airy Chinese lamps, and colorful garlands have a value of self-evident truth in Asiatic nations. In Western nations, people tend to look at them with a critical eye as a "childish form of expression." All of these things are extremely playful and, seen in a sober light, quite without any practical use. They simply give us joy. The color, which is usually red, also stimulates cheerfulness and high spirits.

However, one important exception should be noted here: If roof beams are decorated with garlands, this is intended to ease the pressure coming from the ceiling.

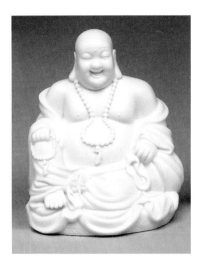

Buddha

Buddha figures are found in almost every household in Asia. The Chinese Buddha is known elsewhere as the Happy Buddha since he embodies not only wisdom but also abundance, wealth, and infinite luck. His inner smile is so strong that it radiates throughout his entire face. The Happy Buddha always wears not only a prayer chain but also brings abundance and both inner and outer wealth to people in bags and mugs.

China also has a wonderful culture of porcelain, so it isn't surprising that the Buddha statues are frequently made of white porcelain.

Dolphin

When dolphins are happy, they jump out of the water and enchant us with their elegant and supple nature. One single dolphin, or even an entire group of dolphins, is not a symbol of partnership like a pair. Instead, it (or all of them) embodies the great treasure of joy in life. For people overburdened with stress and responsibility, reconnecting with playfulness and fun is more important than ever. (For further information about dolphins, please see page 20.)

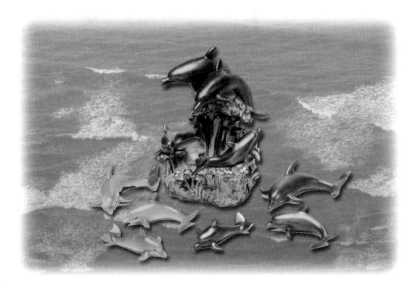

Loving—playful—full of joy in life: Dolphins can impart wonderful feelings to us. All of us can use some support in Zone 7 (Joy in Life). We are frequently so serious and caught up in our tasks that we forget what life and joy in life actually mean.

Dragon

No animal is as closely associated with Chinese philosophy and culture as the dragon. Whether on towels, mugs, and bowls, clothing or decorations, it is found everywhere. On the Chinese New Year, entire groups of people slip as a long column into a giant dragon costume so that this mystic animal can parade through the streets in its entire size.

Every individual has a personal dragon that, similar to a guardian angel, is there for that human being and watches over him or her. In everyday life, the left side of the body takes the position of the dragon. After death, according to a 2000-year-old legend, the soul of the deceased is carried to the higher spheres on the back of the dragon so that it can happily continue its life.

In feng shui, the dragon is the animal of the east, corresponding with the element of wood and the color green. The east is the direction in which dreams can be turned into reality. Who of us hasn't had dreams that would we like to turn into reality?

Lucky dragons, which are displayed in pairs, can be placed anywhere in the home. They help optimize any of the zones.

However, the power of the dragon can best unfold in the east. When the dragon is also connected with the energy of the rising sun, its effect reaches its zenith. Window pictures that contain a crystal together with a dragon motif and hung in a window facing east are the maximum connection of power from the

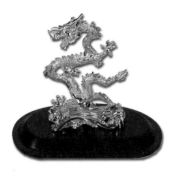

east. They allow great deeds to grow and also give us the necessary ambition to achieve our goals. A young dragon provides us with the necessary impetus; an old, wise dragon watches over us and our plans in a serene manner so that we are protected against harm or thoughtless actions.

Dragon Tears

The greatest jewel that a human being can find on earth from a dragon, according to ancient Chinese legends, is the seed of a dragon. However, since this is a very rare occurrence, a person who has found dragon seed would not let on in the least that he is in possession of this treasure. However, the tears of joy that are cried by dragons when they look down from the high clouds and see that we are happy and content are found somewhat more frequently. On the way from heaven to earth, these tears solidify into crystals.

Dragon tears are enormous, powerful feng shui crystals. Their four tips fling the energy in all four directions and give us feelings of joy, love, and strength. Above all, because of their powerful appearance, they protect people and their rooms from negative influences and keep the good energy in the house. You can hang dragon tears in all of the windows, irrespective of whether they face east, west, south, or north. Since their long axis triggers an active stream of energy similar to that from the healing tip of quartz crystals, they are practically predestined for all "dead corners." If you have enough knowledge on how to do this, you can also use the dragon

tears for charging the bodily energies.

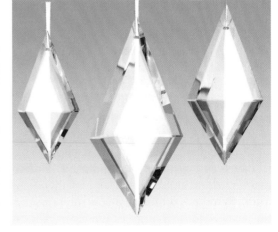

A dragon tear hung in the window is a most effective way to stop energy from passing through it. It has the effect of a sword thrown into the earth from the heavens that blocks the path of escaping energy. If the door and window or two windows face each other, one medium-sized dragon tear should suffice to stop the loss of energy.

Unicorn

In the West, the unicorn is a major symbol of magic. It is always snow-white here, so the magical powers that the unicorn symbolizes are also always white and light. In our culture, the unicorn is kind, loving, wise, and pure. Its deeds are noble and well-considered.

In Asia, the unicorn has a similar meaning, although the unicorn in China sometimes has a black coat. However, this has the following background story: Many years ago, when the country was ruled by dynasties and the emperors, the emperor's horse was the noblest and most beautiful in the entire land. Hundreds of carvings and pictures were made of this most noble (often black) horse of its era. The more distant the possibilities of actually seeing this horse in person or even touching it, the more beautiful, white, and noble it became in the stories. This continued until it was so glorified that it could no longer be a creature of this world. The animal then became mystical and was said to have supernatural abilities. The eight immortals (eight people with special, supernatural abilities) all have a symbol through which they can be recognized, and the emperor's horse became the most recognizable horse of all horses because of the horn, the unicorn. Tribes of riders sometimes put artificial horns on their horses as signs of magical power.

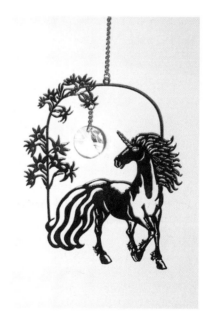

Whether in China or the West, the unicorn is a pure, noble, and glorious creature, which corresponds with the honor of Zone 9 in feng shui. The strength of its character, the power of its body, the wisdom of its mind, and the love and kindness in its heart are the source of glory, honor, admiration, and awe.

Many people perform outstanding work but simply do not receive the recognition due to them from their fellow human beings. Someone who has done something wonderful deserves to be proud of it. But if a person is disregarded, rejected, or even deceived, or has his ideas stolen and others take the credit for his achievements—this person will lose an extreme amount of power and joy, will be frustrated, and ultimately humiliated and injured.

If you feel overlooked in life and do not receive the recognition that is due to you, you can achieve many good things for yourself by strengthening Zone 9. At the same time, it is important to take a critical look with open eyes at the home in terms of Zones 9, 3, and 2. The workplace should also be more closely examined on the basis of the respective zones. A unicorn (illustrated here as a window picture) will not only bring you closer to glory and honor, but also has the effect of an invisible bond between it and you that hardly anyone will risk separating.

Fans

If you have ever been on vacation in Spain, you will know that energies can be distributed and changed with fans. Yet, the circulating energy in the living areas also reacts to the wavy form of the fan's edge and the conducting paths of the inner stays. In Asia, fan culture is highly developed and diversified, ranging from decorative fans and carved fragrant sandalwood fans to battle fans that are dangerous and can even be deadly weapons.

The diversion of energies by using fans is part of the high school of feng shui since there is also an invisible mirror image emanating from the pivotal point that must be included. Like flutes, fans also trigger a cooling, clarifying force.

Flutes

Like an open pair of scissors, two bamboo flutes above the entrance blow away (or cut away) the bad energy that attempts to enter the house. (Since hanging up an open pair of scissors looks quite silly, consider this comment to just be for information purposes.) An additional function of the flutes is to cool the forces. The hotter and stickier the climate, the more we long for a bit of fresh air. In more northerly latitudes, flutes are useful when life demands a certain clarification. When feelings become heated, the flute is one of the things used in feng shui to support a "cool head." When you hang up a flute (normally above the entrance),

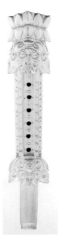

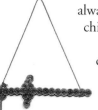

always be sure that the mouthpiece hangs downward so that the light chi can rise upward.

The coin sword (illustrated to the left) is a further variation for cutting through Sha (negative) energy.

Frog

The three-legged frog is a valiant provider of good energy in the material sense. In the early and late morning, it is placed with its eyes looking to the east or southeast so that it can capture the vibration of money's fresh and active energy. The best place for it to sit is on the windowsill where it can look directly (never diagonally) out of the window. In the afternoon, it is turned 180 degrees so that it can "spit" the captured wealth into the home for the remaining hours of the day, giving it to the people who live there.

(In the Asiatic region, spitting and burping are considered a sign of fullness, for "more than enough," and therefore have a very positive meaning.)

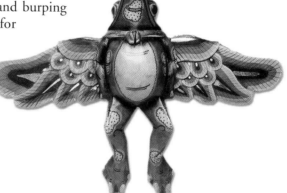

The frog that captures wealth doesn't always have just three legs. This frog from Bali has all four legs, but he has been given wings to make him a "wealth-catcher."

Luck likes to come into a house where a good mood prevails.

— Japanese saying —

The Three Wise Men: Fuk, Luk, and Sau

The three wise men Fuk, Luk, and Sau are very popular messengers of kindness and peace. They radiate boundless inner harmony and great warmth. In their hands, they bear a walking staff (Fuk) as the symbol of infinity, a fruit bowl (Luk) as the symbol for abundance, and a paper scroll (Sau) as the symbol of knowledge. Popular locations for them are the Zones 2 (Relationship) and 4 (Wealth), as well in an accompanying role next to the house altars that are frequently found in China. Additional good locations are Zones 5 (Health) and 6 (Helpful Friends).

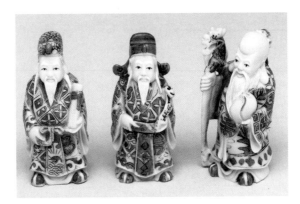

Currency Notes

The 10,000-China-Dollar bills printed by the Hell Bank are the currency of evil spirits. In order to appease them, these bills (20 of them cost about $1.50 or $2.00) are burned. However, this custom is not widespread outside of Asia.

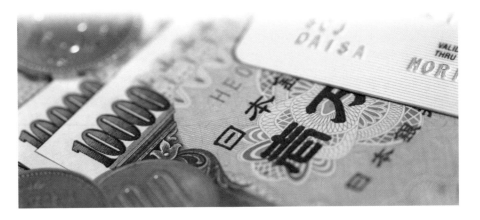

Gnomes and Goblins

Gnomes and goblins are tiny beings who live in the meadows and forests. They frequently draw attention to themselves through their pranks and mischief. Like the angels, gnomes are spiritual beings whose presence we can sometimes sense or feel. They remain concealed from many people for an entire lifetime and are therefore quickly banned to the world of the fairytale and fable by the rational mind. Anyone who is familiar with them knows that they like to accompany human beings and draw attention to themselves by pinching, pricking, and pulling on hair. Their heads are always full of pranks, and they are a spirited folk. There are also many gnomes and goblins in Asia. Some stories tell of very tiny humans or small beings.

Zone 7 in feng shui represents joy in life and contains a great opportunity for adults to forget responsibility, their sense of obligation, and the seriousness of life for a moment. When, like children, we are simply allowed to forget time as we play and just have fun while being together in a friendly way, then we also become like little elves or trolls who enjoy life free of all compulsions and duties.

There are times when we need someone in life who tells us that we should relax, that life is more than seriousness and a sense of duty, that we have created many of our compulsions ourselves, and that there is also wit, laughter, and fun. A gnome in Zone 7 reminds us not to ignore our inner child but to let him or her live and thrive.

Gnomes are associated with the elements of earth and metal. Since they live in little caves in the ground at night, they are said to know about the treasures of the earth, the stones, and the minerals. They are the guardians of caves and watch over mining. As impish as they may act above the ground, they watch over people who are beneath the earth's surface in a protective way.

Golden Fruits

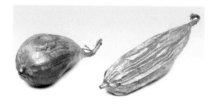

Not only are golden fruits a sign of wealth, they also symbolize oversupply: that there is "more than enough." According to the location and zone, they mean an abundance of material things, of love, of feelings, of inner knowledge, or joy in life. Golden fruits should basically be made of metal (gold-plated brass) so that their ideological significance is directly connected with their effective weight. However, when some type of deficit (tight finances, unfulfilled relationships, etc.) already exists, golden fruits can trigger additional tensions. So use them carefully.

I Ching Signs

In Asia, thousands of people toss their I Ching sticks in front of the temples, sometimes every week, in order to receive advice and help. Feng shui also places much value on the *I Ching, the Book of Changes*. In China, the feng shui masters use it to calculate the appropriate first names for newborns. The parents then choose the name on the list (usually 5 to 10) that most appeals to them. In this manner, the newborn receives a first name promising a happy and successful life and harmonizing with the date of birth and the last name.

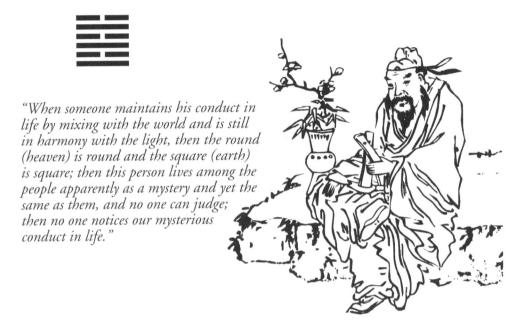

"When someone maintains his conduct in life by mixing with the world and is still in harmony with the light, then the round (heaven) is round and the square (earth) is square; then this person lives among the people apparently as a mystery and yet the same as them, and no one can judge; then no one notices our mysterious conduct in life."

Jade

The opal is inseparably connected with Australia, the amethyst with Brazil, and the jade with China. Chinese stone carvings, which are made of the very best jade whenever possible—the brilliant green Burma or imperial jade—are so perfect and filigreed that we can only stand in front of these works in astonishment and admiration. Whether dragons, Buddhas with flowing robes, or ornamental jars, the high art of stone carving has no boundaries.

Numerous jade disks with two dragons carved on them have been found at excavation sites (mainly tombs). The souls of the deceased were accompanied on their journeys into the higher sphere by jade and protected by the dragons. This

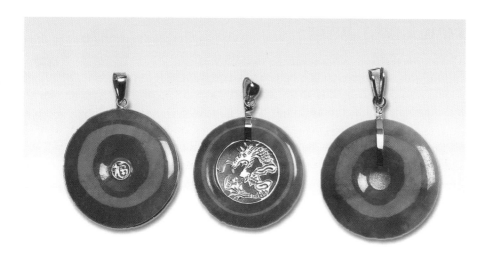

is probably the origin of why jade is also called the "stone of the traveler," even up to the present date. Jade is still a very desired protective stone that many people take along in their pockets, wallets, or naturally as pendants on journeys and in everyday life.

In ancient times, jade was not considered a normal stone. It was a synonym for the seed of the dragon that had turned to stone. For the Chinese, jade is permeated with heavenly power and energy that protects those who carry it with them.

A pendant of beautiful Burmese jade (as illustrated above) protects and strengthens the person who wears it. If you don't want to wear the pendant around your neck, you can tie a little red ribbon to it and carry it with you in your pocket. People sometimes also pinch off the voluminous loop with pliers and give this bringer of good luck and protection a new home in their wallets.

There are also so-called jade crystals available as rainbow crystals. The greenish crystal glass spreads its protective powers over the home and its occupants.

Four-Leaf Clover

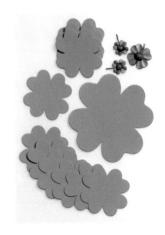

The four-leaf clover is a good-luck symbol in our culture with which everyone is familiar. There are people who constantly find them, and then there are others, like this author, who have never found a single one.

However, regardless of whether a four-leaf clover has been painted or was born in nature, they both bear the same good luck within themselves. The four-leaf clover is a very striking symbol of luck in our culture since it corresponds to four hearts beating in all four directions and uniting at the center (the parallel to the development of the Pa Kua and the five elements cannot be overlooked here). In Chinese symbolism, the cloverleaf has no larger significance. However, the fascination with the four heart-shaped leaves also sparks interest in the Far East.

Cactus

According to the basic rules of feng shui, the cactus is actually a completely unsuitable plant. However, in the Asiatic region there are also no rules without exceptions and the cactus is one of these numerous examples.

Like hardly any other plant, the cactus has the ability to store water. Water, in turn, means wealth. So cacti are a type of "wealth storage." The spines of the cactus symbolize an army of little knives (element of metal) that successfully defend the wealth.

Cacti are best placed on the windowsill so that the negative energy attempting to penetrate from the outside can also be warded off by the spines. If a cactus blooms, then blossoming wealth can also be expected.

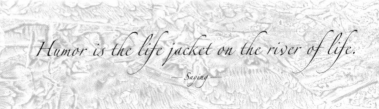

Humor is the life jacket on the river of life.

Saying

Firecrackers

When purchasing property or digging the first spade, or on the Chinese New Year, at every festival, procession, parade, and even during burials at the cemetery, in China evil spirits are driven away with firecrackers. The uninvited guests are dispatched in a noisy and explosive way so that they may disappear forever.

Since firecrackers can cause damage in a home, mock-ups in which the cardboard rolls are empty are also available. In the same way that we can't tell at first glance whether a powder snake is real or not, neither can the evil spirits.

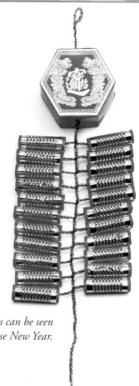

Firecracker mock-up as can be seen everywhere during the Chinese New Year.

Crystals

Feng shui crystals (also called rainbow crystals) are by far the article that is most frequently used in feng shui. They possess two aspects that make them so totally interesting:

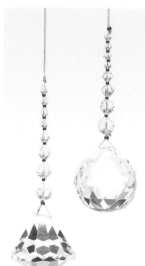

Crystals attract the good energy into a room.

Crystals inhibit the harmful energy that moves within a room.

There is no other feng shui remedy that is so popular for the wrong reasons (namely just the rainbow) and desired like the crystals: When a crystal hangs in the window and the sun shines on it, the glass breaks up the sunbeam into its seven spectral colors and a rainbow is created. These beautiful iridescent splashes of color are what take our hearts by storm and let us completely forget what is actually happening—and what occurs on the secret and invisible level:

When the sun shines into a room, the carpet shows us very clearly how far the sunbeams extend into the area. On the side where the sun shines, the

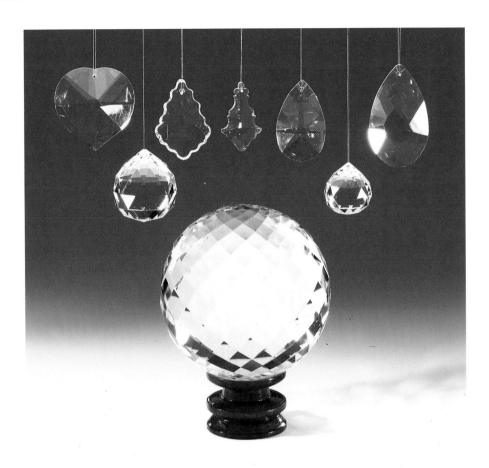

floor is light. The area not reached by the sunshine is distinctly darker. With the support of the rainbow crystals, we can draw this powerful and constructive energy of the sun into the farthest corners of the room.

When the sunbeam hits the crystal, it is caught and opens up in its seven colors. These are then diverted and begin the journey into the room at a completely new angle. So the sun's energy no longer radiates diagonally toward the floor. Instead, depending upon where and how the crystal hangs, it continues to the wall, through the door into the hallway, into the dead corners and nooks, under the ceiling, and wherever you would like to have it.

The secret of the rainbow crystal is not that it creates rainbows but that the chi of the sun is extended by several yards, many times the normal distance, into the room through the ray of sunshine.

56

If the door and window (which may even mean two windows) face each other, the energy will flow unimpeded through the opening into the room. So the room simply cannot become powerful enough on its own. There are various possibilities for catching the exiting energy at the windows and sending it on an "extra round" through the room. The best and most decorative possibilities are: window pictures, mini rose globes (in flowerpots), mobiles, chimes, and naturally the feng shui crystals. By hanging these objects, you can decrease the flight of energy from your rooms.

There seems to be much confusion about the structure of rainbow crystals since all of the qualities are deceptively similar to the naked eye. However, the crystal serves as a transformer and means of conveyance, passing on the sun's energy either in a heavy and placid manner or in a light and airy way.

There is quartz crystal, crystal glass, and lead crystal. Fundamentally, quartz crystal is the best quality, but glass-clear crystals are rare in nature. With a diameter of 1 1/2 to 2 inches, cut spheres cost a small fortune when they are genuine. The cheaper quartz crystal variation is made by a 100% technical procedure with pressure, binding agents, and quartz-crystal dust. I personally find these to be absolutely unsatisfactory for feng shui purposes.

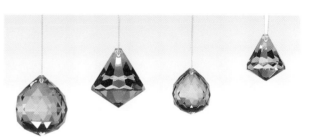

Lead crystal, as the name already says, contains a 20 to 30 percent proportion of lead. These lead crystals are also not appropriate to hang in the window for feng shui purposes. While this lead content makes no difference in beautiful decorative items, bowls, and other forms of lead crystal, we don't hang these bowls and figurines in the window either. They have a completely different purpose, for which they are perfectly suited. However, in terms of feng shui crystals, the means of conveyance is important for extending the sun's energy. (Incidentally, lead crystal has only been known in China since the beginning of the 20th Century and many Chinese find it incomprehensible that lead crystal or pressed quartz crystal could be hung in the window for feng shui purposes.)

Crystal glass, in as far as it is polished and not poured, is the next best solution after pure quartz crystal because the glass is pure and has a high, light vibration. Since the price for crystal glass, according to size, is about 20 to 500 percent cheaper than naturally grown, pure quartz crystal, I clearly prefer working exclusively with crystal glass:

Rainbow crystals with a special wave cut (element of water) are ideal mediators for barred windows since they create a transition from the hard to the soft. Windows with large metal projecting structures as plant holders are frequently

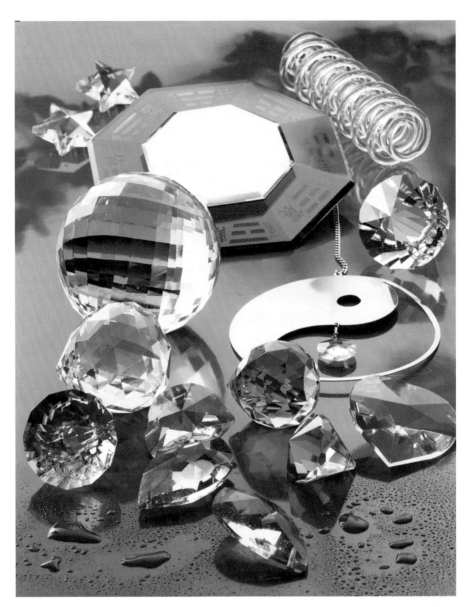

found in rural areas of Europe, but cities tend to have cellar and ground floor windows that are barred.

It is very easy to clean the crystal pendants. Wash them like normal glass and then dry them. Nylon thread (fishing line) is recommended for the least obvious way to hang them up. This nylon thread can even be attached to the curtain rails. But please be sure that the crystal doesn't hit against the window when it opens so that no damage occurs.

Feng shui crystals can be placed in areas other than the window since they also help the "infamous" dead corners. Every apartment and every house has these zones, which we can recognize because the corner beneath the ceiling turns darker than the rest of the wall in the course of passing years. The spent air accumulates here and dust also likes to collect at this point.

However, the crystal needs some support in order to animate dead corners, which can be provided by colors. If a crystal is muted with an iridescent coating (fairy skin), its surface can also be induced to shine with artificial light. These feng shui crystals are "active at night" and, when the lights are turned on in the evening, they bring the occupant much good chi. There is only one variation for making the dead corners shine even during the day: by placing mirrors precisely in the spots where they can redirect the sunbeams to these zones.

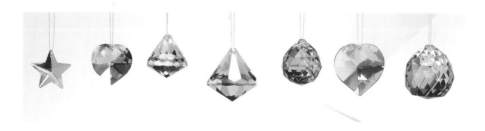

The colored feng shui pendants are available in the colors of green and violet as crystal-glass pendants. The green crystals are associated with jade and the power of the East with the energies of growth and creativity. New beginnings, hope, and protection are symbols from the jade crystal. Violet crystals are mentioned in fairy magic and are the mediator between the lilac (same attributes as above) and red, the power of fire and love. They assume the role of heralds of feelings, emotions, tenderness, and the inner smile.

Please observe the following technical information: Glass can help spark a fire. This also applies to your glasses placed on the dashboard of the car, a glass table close to a window, or a feng shui crystal. Easily inflammable materials can catch fire when there is much solar radiation and close proximity to glass. If you are gone during a summer vacation or have windows facing south, please be sure that the sun does not shine directly on crystals or other glass objects.

Balls

Balls, mainly crystal balls, are associated with a very old tradition. Wherever they appear in the world, people call them "stones of power." Their use as fortune-telling and prophecy balls naturally further intensifies their claim to this title: In Asia, crystal balls are also considered the symbol of eternity since such a sphere has neither a beginning nor an end. It is even more significant than the circle since it also includes the third dimension of depth.

Crystal balls always serve one purpose: harmonization. In the process, it doesn't matter whether this concerns the flow of energy that needs to be calmed (across from the door/window) or emotional/mental imbalances. Just like the Yin Yang symbol, the ball is also a "universal symbol" for harmonizing imbalances.

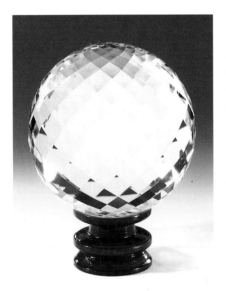

The Wealth Ball

As in so many objects, people naturally attempt to improve the perfect in the shape of the ball. Astonishingly, there is actually an intensified form of the ball. Although a round ball with a flat surface can divert the flow of energy, it cannot change the amount and strength of the energy. By connecting two universal symbols (Yin Yang and ball), a new ball is created that not only harmonizes the flow of energy but also decisively influences its strength. In place of the Sha energy that passes through the home with the power of a jet of water, the Yin Yang ball initiates an atomizing process. Although the negative energy is still present, it is so diffused and dispersed that it no longer has any effective power. So there is no longer anything blocking its effective transformation into chi energy.

In order to perfect every detail of the Yin Yang ball, the number of cuts are also calculated according to numerology. A Yin Yang ball is cut with 384 sides so that the I Ching (64 hexagrams), astrology (12 signs), and time (12 months) can be divided into the number of sides. The Pa Kua, the magical square of feng shui, is also contained in the Yin Yang ball. The cross sum of both the Yin Yang ball and the Pa Kua is the number 15.

In addition to the "technical attributes" explained above, the Yin Yang ball has a very special charm. Its dispersive character has a liberating effect and triggers the inner wealth within us: feelings of contentment, inner peace, and happiness. In stores that display the Yin Yang ball as decoration, the wealth even reaches the cash register. Good fortune is infectious and can be divided endlessly!

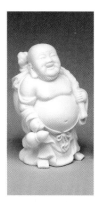

Mug and Bag

Mugs or bags filled to bursting are often found depicted on numerous amulets, statues, or illustrations. Their meaning is abundance, wealth, and prosperity.

The Buddha frequently personally brings the wealth with him, creating the connection between inner and outer wealth in style. Every zone that requires more abundance and weight can be activated by these symbols.

Kwan-Yin

Kwan-Yin ("born from the lotus") is the Queen of Heaven, the patron saint of women, similar to the Mother of God in the West. The Chinese also honor her as the "female Buddha." She is the *Mother of All 10,000 Things*, and exudes gentleness and deep wisdom.

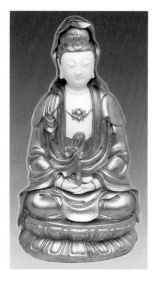

A Kwan-Yin statue in Zone 2 (Relationship) activates the feminine and gentle energies. In addition, it has a very good effect in Zone 6 (Helpful Friends) because this area also represents the source of mental inspiration.

Luo Pan

The Luo Pan is primarily the tool of feng shui consultants who used the Compass School methods, the Eight House methods, or the Flying Star. Although

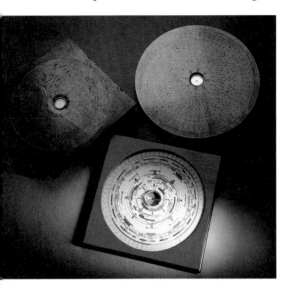

a tool is never better than its user, even a good specialist won't get very far with a poor tool. Logically enough, the traditional Luo Pans from China have Chinese lettering on them. This makes them unsuitable as a serious work instrument for those of us who do not master the Chinese language. Fortunately, beautiful and absolutely precise Luo Pans with plates in English are now available.

The Luo Pan contains all of the possibilities of life, all of the elements, all of the directions, all of the astrological signs, etc. In this light, it isn't surprising that the Luo Pan is very popular as a decorative article in China since it contains the sum of all possibilities.

Tape Measures

Not only colors, forms, elements, and directions are interpreted in feng shui, but the "measure of all things" also has an influence. A new section begins every 2.12 inches and after eight sections = 16.93 inches = one Chinese foot), the cycle begins over again.

Section 1	00.00—02.12 inches	very positive
Section 2	02.13—04.23 inches	negative
Section 3	04.24—06.35 inches	very negative
Section 4	06.36—08.46 inches	very positive
Section 5	08.47—10.58 inches	positive
Section 6	10.59—12.70 inches	very negative
Section 7	12.71—14.81 inches	negative
Section 8	14.82—16.93 inches	positive

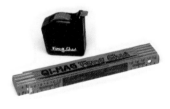

It is reported that these measurements were calculated on the basis of the I Ching. Yet, it is astonishing how many Chinese masters completely ignore these measurements and do not integrate them into their computations. It may well be that these are Japanese feng shui measurements or those of measuring units from other Asian countries that flowed together in the 20th Century. However, there is also the possibility that this is a "modern phenomena." Or it may be nearly forgotten knowledge that was spread in a regional and very well-guarded manner and has now been passed on to a larger public.

Minerals

Minerals in their natural state possess an extremely strong and powerful vibration of their own. Groups of crystals not only radiate the power of depth but also disperse the negative energy that likes to collect in corners and dead zones. A little piece quartz crystal in a corner area can work genuine wonders. If you clean your minerals under flowing water on a regular basis, they will be your friends for life.

Mobiles

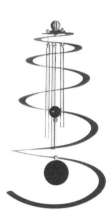

In contrast to Chinese lanterns and garlands, we "Westerners" have no problem getting accustomed to mobiles. Modern designs and attractive forms are much more in keeping with our culture than red Chinese lanterns or colorful garlands.

Mobiles, garlands, chimes, and colorful ribbons are all nourished by the same energy and brought to life by the wind. In China, the wind is the father of many good airs: wealth, abundance, and luck. So mobiles that are breathed on by the wind are a symbol of life, wealth, and luck.

Monks

Monks devote their lives to the study of inner values. But the rest of us, who are sometimes caught up in a very stressful daily routine or profession, can at best dedicate ourselves to advancing the education of our minds in the evening or on the weekend. Yet, we are often already so exhausted at these times that there isn't

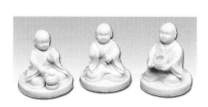

much opportunity for meditation, education, and inner training. So we remain a kind of "little monk" for our entire lives. While the sculptures of the great masters and sages symbolize the perfection of mental/spiritual development, the child monks are a loving self-depiction of our own personality on the path to the great goal. Ideal locations are Zone 8 (Knowledge), Zone 3 (Family), as well as Zone 4 (Wealth/Inner Wealth).

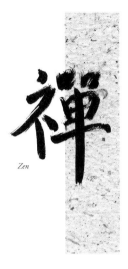

Zen

Ox and Farmer

The story of the farmer who chases after his runaway ox until he learns to take the path with it is one of the very renowned philosophical stories of Asia. The Ox Story (as it is commonly called) is a journey through 10 steps to enlightenment and has an extremely high level of spiritual importance. In case you are not familiar with this story and are interested in Asian philosophy, I can warmly recommend that you read it. The 10th step (the farmer rides home on the back of the ox and plays a flute) is a very widespread symbol in Asia for success on the foundation of intelligent thoughts and actions. (Location: Zone 9 = Fame.)

Pagoda

The pagoda is a temple of knowledge and wisdom, of peace and silence. The pagoda is a place of power and corresponds with Zone 8 (Mountain) in feng shui. An illustration of a pagoda symbolizes the inner center, the power of the mind, as well as active inner growth. A person who knows more or is knowledgeable stands firm like a mountain or a pagoda and cannot be shaken by anything. The gently

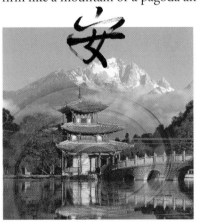

sloping roof of a pagoda, upon which the wind rises to the heavens, is the connection to the divine force.

If a bridge runs across the calm water of a lake to the temple of knowledge, the powers of the heavens are connected with the depth of the water.

This image symbolizes the path of wisdom.

The pagoda is perfectly oriented in terms of the 5 animals. (Mountain behind, hills to the right and left, lake in front)

Pa Kau Mirror

The Pa Kau mirror and rainbow crystals are now so widespread that they have already been called the "aspirin of feng shui."

However, just like the rainbow crystals serve as conveyance and extension paths for chi energy and place corresponding demands on the materials, the Pa Kau mirror also requires certain rules that are irrevocable.

In abstract and technical terms, a Pa Kau mirror is an octagonal mirror that has eight trigrams in the order of the "prenatal heavens."

In the "prenatal (early) heavens," the earth is below, the sky is above, and we human beings— when we look in the mirror—are in the middle. All tools of life (trigrams) are arranged around the mirror in a perfectly harmonious manner. This order corresponds with the origin, with not acting, with true and absolute harmony. This is the beginning and also the destination.

In the teaching of feng shui itself, a different order is used for dividing the nine sectors, which is the post-natal (later) heavens. Here the individual trigrams interact with each other. They mutually trigger movement and change, just as in our everyday routine and daily lives. Despite this, we all have the desire to find peace and harmony, meaning the "prenatal heavens." And we find these origins in the Pa Kau mirror.

NOTE: If an octagonal mirror has absolutely no lettering, then it cannot represent either one or the other form of change. The mirror then has virtually no message. No Chinese person would ever elevate an octagonal mirror without inscriptions to the value of a Pa Kau mirror.

However, the type of inscription is also subject to distinct rules and laws. Even in very old writings, the rule was that a mirror should never be written on directly since there were no waterproof felt pens or adhesive paint. As a result, the trigrams would have either been carved or scratched into the mirror. However, this would have destroyed the compact nature of the glass. So people decided to only write on the reverse side of mirrors. A wooden frame was later built around the mirror, which could now have the trigrams painted

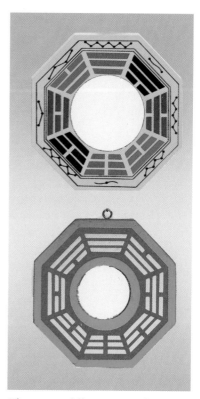

There are two different versions of traditional Pa Kau mirrors in this picture. The red-green wooden mirror is the standard mirror from China, but usually of very poor quality. The yellow mirror is an additional, quite useful variation that has better workmanship.

onto it. Only since the invention of modern laser technology has it been possible to engrave mirrors from the reverse side without influencing the glass in the front. So Pa Kau mirrors made according to all the rules of the ancient sages have only been available for the past few years.

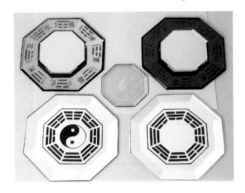

The five mirrors illustrated here have been inscribed on the reverse side with the most modern technology and therefore correspond with the original standards.

These mirrors are available in three variations: straight, concave, and convex.

Straight mirrors always attract the energy found in the mirror image. This naturally also applies to all "normal mirrors" that we have in the house (bathroom, wardrobe, bedroom, etc.) It is therefore very useful to first check to see what is facing the mirror and whether this energy is worth doubling. No matter where it is, a straight mirror always demands something beautiful facing it. You can achieve this with pictures, healthy and blossoming plants, or a joyful symbol or object. Thanks to an attractive mirror image, you can create an extremely high flow of good energy that will spread throughout the entire room in the course of time.

Concave mirrors are like little bowls in which good energy can be collected. When you place a bowl in the sink and turn on the tap, water will collect in it. The same principle applies to the concave mirror, which also corresponds with the principle for the straight mirror: whatever is facing the mirror will determine what it collects. There is truly a difference between whether it draws in the power of a blossoming tree or the dull facade color of the neighbor's house. In Hong Kong, where many people live in skyscrapers, people like to place mirrors (straight and concave forms) on the windowsills in order to attract the powerful energy of the heavens and with it the good spirits, which are invited into the home. This naturally functions not only in skyscrapers, but wherever the sky can be reflected in the mirror (see ill., page 67, above).

Convex mirrors have a completely different function than the straight and concave ones. They are meant to send back undesired things and energies. If we take the example of the bowl in the sink, we turn the bowl upside down in this variation. Now slightly turn on the tap so that the water flows over the hemisphere. In just the same way, negative energy will flow off and not find a foothold to stay and cause a disruption. If the jet of water is intensified, the water will spray off in all directions. A strong negative energy and any sensitive disorder will then immediately be sent back to its producers. In this way, sharp house edges of neighboring buildings, evil energies from people, lantern masts, and all other forms of emissions are combated. (See ill. page 67, below.)

However, there is also a very special variation here: If the good energy in a room flows away too quickly (example: you would like to keep the creative energy a bit longer in a room), then the good energy is sent on a type of "extra round" thanks to the convex form and the creative impulses circulate longer and more intensely. Since this kind of mirror may look rather funny for Western tastes, it is advisable to put a very small rose globe (about 2 inches in size) in with the indoor plants at the window. (See Rose Globes on pages 32-34.)

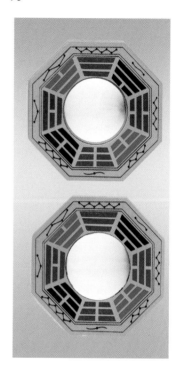

Depending upon the school of feng shui, it is taught that mirrors are to be used in a very sparing or extremely lavish manner. Or that they should be only applied outside or everywhere in general. The reasons for this inconsistency are mainly the geographic differences in the huge country of China. The personal preferences of the individual masters have played an additional, not insignificant role in these discrepancies. Since "major energetic mistakes" can quickly be made within the living area (when the mirror image is wrong), beginners are initially taught to not use any mirrors in interior rooms. During the course of the training, these rules are then generally qualified. If you would like to do something good for yourself, then check all of the mirror images in your home—it's worth doing. Using this careful approach, you can hang up the straight and concave (collecting) Pa Kau mirrors in your home as well.

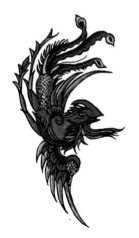

Phoenix

The phoenix is one of the five classic animals of feng shui and embodies the feminine principle.

Together with the dragon, the phoenix embodies the Yin Yang of the heavens. They are the pair of lovers that are connected for all of eternity.

By itself, the phoenix, which has risen out of the ashes, embodies infinity and rebirth. The energy and the power of hope, one of the greatest driving forces of humanity, is represented by the phoenix. The picture of

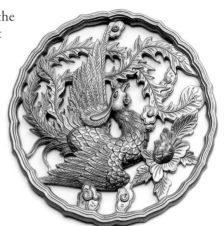

a phoenix gives us human beings the strength to continue, to survive difficult times, and never lose courage. Although this symbol is rarely found in the West, the phoenix is certain to soon reach our latitudes since its message is beautiful and acts like a gentle balsam on our stressed souls.

The colors of the phoenix are red and orange, and its direction is the south.

Rainbows

Rainbows are a wonderful creation of the heavens and enchant us time and again. Even today, it is not possible to bring a rainbow down to earth or find its beginning or its end. Rainbows appear, they fascinate us, and then they simply dissolve again into the vast void.

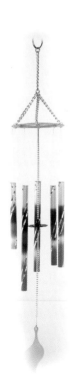

We can only see rainbows when the sun shines into the rain. They are the crowning of two elements connected with each other in a cycle that together produce a new, third energy.

When fire (sun) and water (rain) meet, steam is created on the earth and a rainbow in the heavens. So it isn't surprising in feng shui that rainbows represent every type of connecting and merging. They show us that the impossible is possible and that things happen beyond our rational minds, which we can only accept in amazement.

In ancient China, the rainbow was the bridge between Yin and Yang, the feminine and the masculine. Only in connection with rainbows could the third energy, a new human life, be created.

Rainbows contain the seven spectral colors of light. The more brilliant the colors are, the stronger the new energy can be. This is why chimes in the colors of the rainbow are usually very color intensive and brilliant in feng shui.

The rainbow chimes illustrated here are inexpensive and consists of five tubes that emit a very bright sound. These chimes symbolize the area of our health with a colorfully strong, luminous expressive power, as well as cheerfulness through their bright sound.

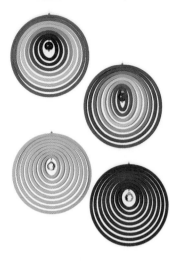

All of the crystals that conjure rainbows into rooms are also bridge-builders between the yin energy and the yang energy.

The same also applies to objects, mobiles, and pictures that are painted in the colors of the rainbow.

Incense Sticks

In Asia, an incense stick accompanies every message to the heavens. Just as the smoke begins to rise up, the message travels on this little cloud. Burning incense is an absolutely obvious gesture directed toward the gods.

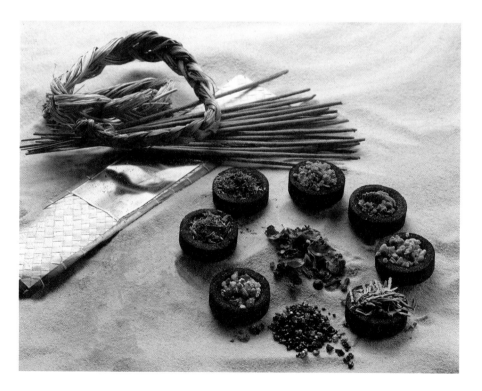

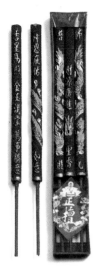

Chinese incense sticks often have a somewhat biting smell for our Western noses. Although we normally only light incense sticks in closed rooms, Asians quite frequently use them in the outdoors and in front of temples. As a result, different mixtures and qualities are required in keeping with the respective situation.

Special prayer incense sticks

Red Stamp

Whether calligraphic works, wall pictures, pictures on scrolls, or cards, there is almost always a little red stamp on the side. Its content, the name of the arts, as well as the place and date, are less spectacular than its power of visual expression. In the West, sealing wax is also red. So the color speaks first, and through it the element of fire, and only then does the message follow. Important things are also always stamped in red.

Tortoise

The tortoise represents one of the five animals of feng shui and embodies protection and security. Its shell protects against all attacks from the north, where an icy and cold wind blows in China—and this breeze isn't very pleasant in other places either.

In everyday life, this "cold attack from the north" is equated with the unprotected back of human beings. The shell of the tortoise is like a warm coat that protects us. However, it is not just the wind that we would like to keep away from us. We need protection and security in many of life's situations. The more protection we need, the more the tortoise becomes a valuable and true friend.

The color of the tortoise is black or blue, and its direction is the north.

(You can find more information about the classifications and nature of the five animals in *The Complete Feng Shui Health Handbook* written by Gerstung/Mehlhase, Lotus Press 2000.)

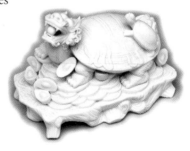

Snake

The snake is also one of the five animals of feng shui and represents the center, tranquillity, and peace. Like the sun that radiates in all directions and warms us, the snake awakens energy and initiative within us and within our fellow human beings.

Whether during tai chi, chi gong, or other practices that awaken the chi, the energy is always collected at the center of the body, the *tantien* (called *hara* by the Japanese), built up, and then passed on to the respective organs and parts of the body.

"There's strength in silence," "everything revolves around the center, "the power is at the center,"—all of these wise words are directly connected with the symbolism of the snake: The colors of the snake are brown, ocher, yellow, and gold. The direction is the center.

Snow Crystals

The snow crystal is a symbol from Japanese feng shui. This extremely filigreed, fragile, and delicate structure can only exist in the present, in the moment of the here and now. The snow crystal, as well as the ice flower, also symbolizes purity and nobility.

In numerous Japanese feature films, the snow falls from heaven and the dying leading man is covered completely with snow flakes and snow crystals in the last act. In this way, vast importance is placed upon the present and neither the past nor the future exist in any form.

In our thoughts, we frequently live in the past or the future, yet our life takes place in the here and now. If we would concentrate all the energy that we invest in past times and future thoughts into the present, we would suddenly have more time and more strength. The course that we set today is the success, the peace, and the inner and outer wealth of tomorrow. The here and now sets the course for our path in life tomorrow. It is a type of master control for our own personal happiness. This is the principle existing within the snow crystals.

Snow crystals are primarily associated with the direction of the north or Zone 1, which represents our path in life and career. However, wherever our thoughts drift off—whether in love, work, health, or joy in life—the snow crystals are the guide back to the path.

The idea of snow crystal and the Zen philosophy at their core are inseparably connected with each other.

Characters

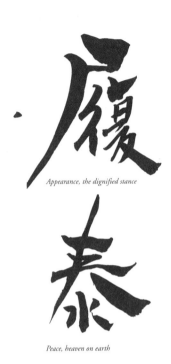

Appearance, the dignified stance

Peace, heaven on earth

Chinese characters are extremely popular balancing tools, guardians, and heralds of strength. The calligraphic writing of a word is normally divided into two processes: The utmost goal of the first is to write it in a beautiful, elegant, and sound manner that is also correct according to all of the guidelines.

Very few people master the second way since the statement of the word is connected with the respective chi energy during the writing. Actually, all of the great masters, whether in feng shui or the martial arts, have catapulted their inner powers to an extremely high level through years of practicing qi gong and related practices. When a master does calligraphy, breathing is always synchronized with the drawing of the lines.

The energy is pushed out through the breath so that the hand remains still. The creation of an energy-charged calligraphic work is always accompanied by hissing, muffled, loud, quiet, or even echoing sounds.

Those of us in the West who cannot read Chinese still feel the difference in the energy. Even on a reproduction, the way in which the character was created remains clearly perceptible.

Good words find their home anywhere. Calligraphic works that have the word "love" or "life" written on them are naturally most advantageous in the partnership zone. However, love knows no boundaries and so there is no wrong location for it. Luck, chi, Tao, peace, and many other beautiful words are naturally universal.

Sun

Feng shui recognizes three main sources that contain the creative power of the chi energy. These are light, fresh air, and warmth. Heat, and with it the feeling of warmth, is most directly stimulated by the sun. When the sun hardly shines during the gray winter months, we feel like someone has taken the elixir of life from us. Whether human being, animal, or plant—we are all tickled by the sun's rays in spring and let ourselves be filled with this pleasant warmth.

The sun gives us strength, energy, and joy in life. As a result, it also indirectly helps our health and inner harmony. A sun in the house is the symbol of all these strengths and the great universal warmth that never fails. In the ancient cultures (and even today in Japan), the sun was always considered feminine and worshipped as the Sun Goddess, as a symbol of universal warmth and love. Later in history, the moon then became the symbol of the feminine and the sun the symbol of masculine energy.

Sun motifs are simple to find. There are countless variations in wood, plastic, metal, large and small, colorful and neutral. We can find the motif of the shining sun on chimes, on the face of clocks, and on bed linens.

We could not exist on this planet without the sun. It lets the plants grow and human beings thrive. According to feng shui, the sun most strongly supports the areas of health (5), joy in life (7), and the zones of wealth (4) and relationship (2). However, other additional zones can be strengthened by the power of the sun. It has a further positive side effect on the path in Life Zone (1) since it makes the first step, the beginning, easier. Independent of the Pa Kua zone, a sun symbol always represents an activation of beneficial energies.

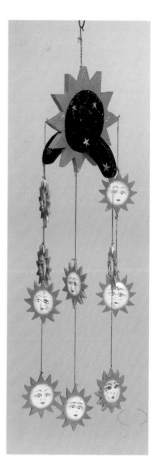

When the rays of the sun touch a crystal in the window, it is as if a second sun begins to shine.

Spirals

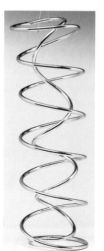

There are currently two types of spirals that are quite familiar and widespread in the West, one type made of crystal glass (pg. 74, above), the other of metal spirals (pg. 73). All kinds of plastic and shiny foil spirals are available, but they tend to be more playful decorative articles than feng shui remedies. These are colorful and fun to look at, which supports our joy in life. Some plastic spirals even have a little motor so that they turn incessantly—which is ideal for awakening the "inner child."

DNS spirals (with a few exceptions) are made of metal and help energize the living and working areas of the home. They have an extremely active effect on the energy household of a room. I consider it quite sensible to not just hang the

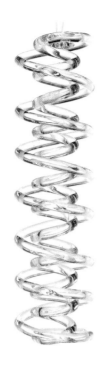

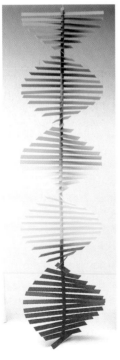

metal spirals up anywhere but always have the right location for them defined by a specialist. Clarifying energies are released by the element of metal, yet these are frequently also associated with a confrontation in the current life situation. A person who too quickly "clears the decks" can "overshoot" the goal, affronting other people and hurting their feelings. Metal spirals are active spirals, which means that they are constantly moving to some degree and turn themselves. DNS spirals are a very effective aid for upgrading zones lacking energy, clarifying life situations, and activating new paths. However, they belong in the hands of specialists.

The crystal-glass spirals behave in a completely different manner. Because of their material, they correspond with the element of water and represent communication and togetherness. Pleasant, constructive conversation and the exchange of feelings and ideas is an important foundation for every relationship, as well as both private and business goals and interests.

Crystal-glass spirals are a symbol of the infinity principle since they have neither a beginning nor an end. This is why the Chinese also have no spirals that just turn to the left or the right. If the outer coil turns to the left, the inner coil automatically turns to the right. The division of an infinite spiral into left and right sections is like first breaking apart the Yin Yang symbol in order to put it back together again. However, if a spiral just has one arm, then the energy form of the spiral that turns to the left corresponds with the yin energy and the feminine, while the spiral turning to the right is associated with the masculine principle, the yang.

The core of every crystal spiral is numerology. Spirals achieve their expressive power and inner dimension through the number of their inner and outer coils. The eight coils in the outer spirals represent the overall influences that human beings encounter in the course of their lives (8 x 8 = 64 = I Ching) and the eight outer zones of the Pa Kua (the center is associated with the inner spirals). The inner spirals with their twelve coils correspond to the human being (twelve astrological signs) and the principle of transience, of time, with which we are inseparably linked.

Crystal spirals are wonderful to hang up in zones with a low flow of energy, in all corners, and also on the ceiling of very tall rooms. They are very fragile, so don't place them in front of an open window. And it also fundamentally isn't sensible to place any remedies, no matter what marvelous qualities they have, directly above the places where people sit or sleep.

The less crystal spirals turn, the closer they are to their core statement: finding the inner center and inner repose. Or, as the TAO says in such a wonderful way:

Acting by not acting.

Tiger

The tiger is also among the five animals of feng shui. It embodies activity, energy, and initiative. Its strength is synonymous with our entire personal spirit of struggling for existence. How we master our lives often depends on our sense of survival, our inner fighting spirit. A tiger retreats, but it never gives up.

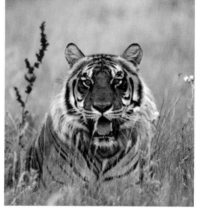

Tiger symbols and drawings with tigers are always an expression of power and strength. They embody the almost untamable and tremendous energy that we each have within us.

Those who carry great plans within themselves and feel impelled to master a task that requires an extreme amount of strength can strengthen themselves with the support of a tiger picture.

The color of the tiger is white, and its direction is the west.

Here is a Chinese saying:

Lure the tiger from the mountains.

Since this is a strategic image, it means neither the mountains nor the tiger but the boundless, explosive power that we can awaken within ourselves in order to do great and important deeds. The ability to "lure the tiger from the mountains" in our fellow human beings is taught and practiced as the high art of strategy.

Door Signs

Door signs and business lettering contain a very important statement. The size, form, colors, material, and location are analyzed in a very precise manner. In Asia, the corporate identity of a company has a much more extensive meaning than in the West since it can determine whether it "sinks or swims." It is therefore not surprising that neither the company boss, nor the owner, nor the graphic artist has the last word about the company logo—but the feng shui master.

In the private sphere, the door sign is analogous in importance to the social position. For "normal mortals," clean, clear, and flawless lettering is sufficient.

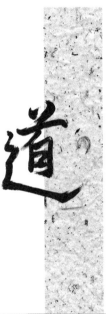

Immortals

The seven (or eight) immortals are personalities that have not only achieved absolute wisdom but also possess supernatural abilities. According to the different versions, these are seven men or seven men and one woman. Although these stories are very widespread in China, Chinese immortals don't have a significant meaning in the West. The Chinese like to place the seven (eight) immortals close to their house altars since these personalities live in the clouds and the heavens, which connect them with the supernatural.

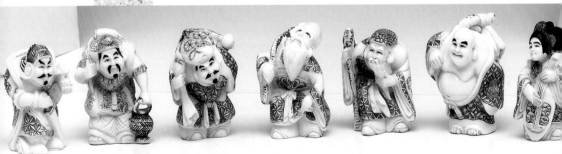

Waterfalls

In feng shui, water is associated with two energies: with communication (element of water) and with money. A large, thundering waterfall therefore corresponds with an unending shower of money, under which many people would like to stand. However, a great deal of caution must be exercised in selecting pictures of waterfalls. For example, what use is the loveliest waterfall when there is no large lake beneath it to collect the shower of money? A simple rule of thumb applies here: one part waterfall, two parts lake. The lake must give the viewer the feeling that it is already deep, wide, and mighty and can absorb at least twice the volume of the waterfall within itself before it passes along the energy.

A waterfall without a lake is like winning at lotto and then immediately receiving a demand for back payment from the IRS. Perhaps a "few drops" will remain in the end but the entire huge blessing was nothing more than a "cash flow."

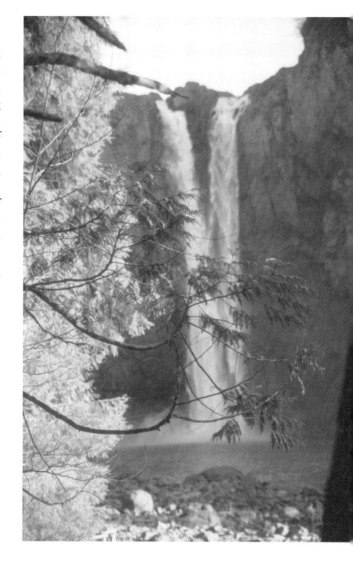

Waterfall pictures are wonder-ful, highly potent, and activating sources of energy that can not only optimize your zone of wealth (4), but also the joy in life (7), path in life (1), health (5), and love (2).

Waterfall pictures are frequently left unframed so that the wealth can flow without limitations, which is basically a perfect situation. However, since paper is somewhat sensitive, the colors in unframed pictures can become faded and yellowed and the edges and sides frayed. But since picture frames made of glass, in a blue or black color correspond with the element of water, this limitation only means a repetition of the picture.

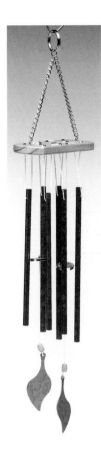

Chimes

Wind chimes, also called magic bells, are among the most frequently used feng shui cures. They are the heralds of two wonderful messages:

cheerfulness and brightness (through the sound) and
life (that the wind breathes into the tubes).

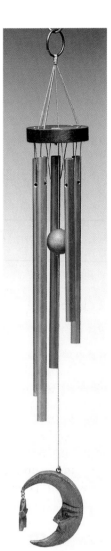

People like to hang wind chimes and magic bells above entrance doors. This is a type of feng shui "alarm system." If the door is opened, they make a sound. In the garden or on the balcony, ringing wind chimes are always a sign of life and information to uninvited guests that someone lives in the house or apartment.

There are just a few easily understood instructions to observe when hanging up wind chimes. When the wind chimes are located above the door, they do not sound because of the contact with the door instead of the wind. It is very important that just a gentle contact occurs since the tubes will otherwise crash against each other and the wind chimes don't sound but clatter and clank. The same also applies to spirals, lamps, crystals, and much more: nothing should be placed directly above the heads and the ceiling should be free of dangling objects (guillotine effect) above the sleeping area. In the garden or on the balcony, how brightly or strongly the wind chimes move is a matter of the wind strength. The same thing applies here: a gentle ringing is more pleasant than a "frenzied sound."

The number of tubes naturally has a meaning as well. However, there are some very astonishing stories in circulation about this matter. Fortunately, there is no "wrong number of tubes." Wind chimes with three tubes or ornaments are more frequently played by hand, wealth is awakened by those with four tubes (which is the most difficult number), the connection to the inner center and health is the main aspect with five tubes, the heavenly helpers are invited with six tubes, and the joy in life is kissed awake by seven tubes. Recently, people have started discussing whether hollow or filled tubes are better. You can decide this for yourself with listening to your inner voice. Listen to the tone and let your eyes play a role in making the decision.

Many Chinese amulets have little bells attached to them so that they come to life through the wind and develop their power.

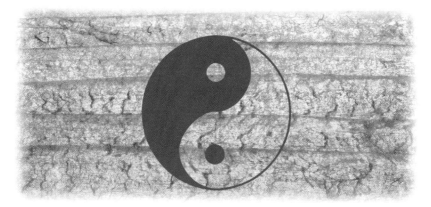

Yin Yang

The Yin Yang symbol is certainly the best known of all Chinese symbols. Two equally strong twin forces are so inseparably united into a circle that neither could exist without the other (or can only exist at all thanks to the other). Yin (which literally means: the shaded)and yang (which literally means: the sunbathed) are in absolute harmony and total balance with each other. Wherever and whenever we leave this inner center in our lives, the yin-yang forces are no longer in harmony.

Anger, annoyance, sadness, pain, stress, frustration, disappointment—almost all of our feelings are either too yin or too yang. The entire range of Chinese medicine (acupuncture, acupressure, etc.), as well as the healing gymnastics of tai chi and chi gong have "the principle of fullness and emptiness" as their basis. When a brick falls on your toe, you have a fullness (even if it was undesired)— which can be counteracted by emptiness or a distribution throughout the entire body. In anger and stress we also collect energies within us that cause an unhealthy fullness. We then have the feeling of bursting inside. Disappointments and exhaustion result in a feeling of emptiness that requires new energy.

The yin and yang forces are constantly in motion within us human beings at all times. They are stimulated and influenced on the one hand by our feelings and on the other hand by our physical condition. The Yin Yang symbol can be used anywhere in order to reinstate balance or achieve harmony.

Depending on the zone, it also has an effect on other areas of life. Whether you are striving for a stronger degree of harmony with a relationship (Zone 2), desire more strength and stability for your health (Zone 5), less stress in your working life (Zones 1 and 9) and more enjoyment of life (Zone 7), or more inner or more outer wealth (Zone 4), the Yin Yang symbol generally helps in every area.

We Are What We Radiate

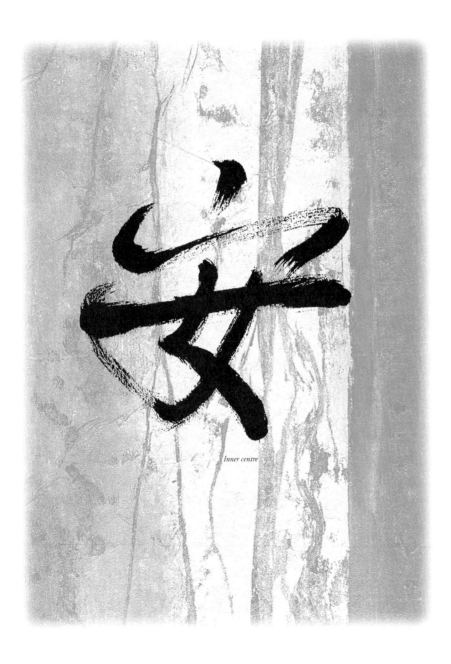

Inner centre

Pictures

Not too long ago, Hollywood let the Titanic sink again. It naturally didn't take long for the related posters and pictures to be hung up in a great variety of homes. The example of the Titanic is one of the best to explain the meaning or content of pictures according to feng shui: The floating ship as a picture is an imposing structure, yet we all know of its sad ending. It is therefore a symbol of a future downfall, an impending tragedy, and not advisable from the perspective of feng shui. On the other hand, there is the picture in which the lovers of the film stand at the front of the ship with outstretched arms—a symbol of eternal love and boundless freedom. However, this picture is also overshadowed by the sad ending. Melancholy, sadness, and wistfulness—all feelings related to the first great pangs of love—are stimulated. It isn't surprising that teenagers feel magically attracted to this picture.

Many people like abstract art or pictures that have no concretely recognizable images on them. Pictures consisting of lines, waves, circles, squares, or dots may have an "top and bottom" in purely theoretical terms. But this is the perspective as seen by the artist. However, there is no rule that an abstract picture can't be turned by 90 degrees or even upside down. I have already given a number of pictures a new perspective and more expressive power by simply turning them. And I'm sure that I am not the only one who has done this: You are certain to have heard that galleries and exhibits of the works of very famous artists have presented the pictures by hanging them the wrong way. This is where the optimists and the pessimists are at odds with each other and feng shui can offer extremely interesting interpretations and explanations about the artist's relationship to the various zones.

Inherited oil paintings are another story since they are usually completely unattractive in terms of their market value. Yet, there is always the possibility that they conceal a great value. Most boring pictures just get dusty in silence on the wall. Go ahead and take down a "landscape in the fog." Take your picture to an expert, who can tell you at first glance whether the painting only has value for your family. If you are artistically talented, you can infuse a sunset into the landscape in the fog (if it is worthless) and pep it up with a cheerful frame.

Pictures aren't "holy cows," although we would like to treat them that way. They radiate a lot of energy into a room—or they take it away. Use your walls for pictures that you like and enjoy. Thanks to their strong colors and visible joy in life, children's pictures exude an enormous amount of chi. The material value of a picture is just secondary in feng shui.

Flowers and Plants

Flowers and plants are a symbol of blossoming love, of strength, vitality, and joy in life, as long as they are healthy and have roots. Various feng shui books disapprove of plants with long, pointed leaves and only approve of those with roundish and oval leaves. I know of many people who have liquidated, disposed of, and

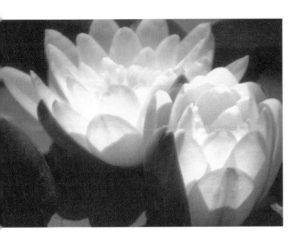

thrown away plants that they had loved for many years as a result of this advice. I think this is very sad and, above all, irresponsible on the part of the authors. We don't have such a great variety of plants in this world that we can despise half of them. The form of the plant leaves represents the elements, and the pointed leaves stand for the element of fire (triangle). Long, thin leaves symbolize the element of metal when they look like little knives or scalpels. However, people who bear the element of earth within themselves are nourished by the element of fire—so triangular leaves would be ideal for them. Those who have the personal element of water are supported by the power of the metal element. However, these two leaf forms require a careful selection for the plant's location so that the energy of the leaves cannot separate or cut the good chi that flows in the room.

Plants need care, attention, and some of our love. They like it when we talk to them and take care of them. Some plants have moved several times with their owners and still enjoy a ripe old age. However, our green friends sometimes look a bit older than they really are. Haggard and exhausted, with thin stems and falling leaves, they become stunted. We put up with them because we are too lazy to get rid of them, and not because we are merciful. Sometimes the age of a plant can be almost read on the layer of dust on its leaves. Replanting, watering, and cleaning them—or supplying some new soil—is usually enough to give a plant fresh courage in life.

Plants are living beings. Like humans, they are not immortal. We assume responsibility for their care the day we acquire them. You can help a sick plant by placing it in Zone 3, Family. In the Family Zone, also called Rotation, it will become active again. If it has enough strength left, it will also regain its health. It is advisable to only place "short-term patients" in the Relationship Zone since the area of relationship will otherwise receive this aura of being sick and tired. However, a brief stay in this zone can be extremely healing and regenerative for a sick plant.

At the center of every floor plan, in the Health Zone, there is usually a lack of the necessary daylight for our green friends to grow powerful and strong, to live and blossom. Consequently, it is sensible to not place any green plants in the center area since they may represent everything but health after a short amount of time there.

Cut flowers can radiate wonderful chi energy. However, this just lasts very briefly. Since they have been separated from their roots, they get weaker by the hour until they let their heads hang and begin to wilt. On festive occasions or simply as a personal touch of delight, flower bouquets and arrangements with cut flowers decorate the dining table. As long as the flowers are fresh and the water is clean and clear, the good chi will be effective. But once the flowers let their heads hang, the breath of life leaves them and they wilt. Now it is time, at the latest, to thin out the bouquet or arrangement and remove the wilted flowers. Many people don't even like to separate from completely wilted flowers because they were a gift from someone very close to them. However, the love and feelings that the flowers represent dwell in the gesture of giving and in the heart: they are not attached to the flowers. So go ahead and throw away the faded roses and wilting bouquets in good time.

Various plants are not only strong contributors of chi, but also possess a deeper symbolism and are accordingly honored and protected.

Jasmine: Symbol of deep, honest friendship and inner beauty

Willow: Grace, devoted and reserved nature, gentleness

Plum: Connection of yin and yang. Fair, clear actions (branches and fruits) in a delicate, fragile, and gentle manner (blossoms)

Lotus: Symbol of infinity and equilibrium of yin-yang energies. Roots under water = immortality and the power from the depths of the curved stem under water = umbilical cord of life
flower above the water = materialization in the light.

Peony: Royal flower and bearer of pure yang energy. It represents fame, wealth, masculinity, and self-realization in the light.

Almond blossom: Symbol of feminine beauty, but also of still and quiet suffering.

Books

Time and again, course participants and clients have told me that they have read something negative in feng shui guides about having an abundance of books. So the advice of storing the books that they have read in the cellar was immediately taken. However, the result was depressing and disappointing for many people.

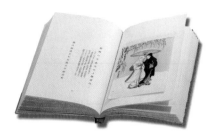

The once splendidly filled shelves are now empty and a feeling of loneliness spreads throughout the living room. These people feel like something very precious has been taken from them. There are many individuals who collect books and like to browse in them now and then. In turn, others read their books from cover to cover and feel enriched by having them around.

In the living room, it is usually "just" a question of the amount of books that creates good or bad feng shui. In this case, the principle of yin and yang, of abundance and emptiness is the basis of all decisions. If the books are piled up so high that not a single spot of space exists anywhere, an excess of abundance has been created and now demands emptiness. Even a bookshelf in the living room demands that at least 15 to 30 percent of the free space be filled with decorative objects or just "nothing at all." Ideal books for the living room are: picture books, reference works, and books with a content that encourages relaxation and well-being.

Some individuals also like to "store" books in the bedroom. However, they are completely out of place here. Since people enjoy reading a few pages in bed at night before they go to sleep, the current book and a handful of others can remain in the bedroom. However, a bookcase directly next to the bed is more than just a strain on the mind that would like to rest at night. Like a hanging lamp directly over the head gives the subconscious mind the feeling of a guillotine in a stand-by position, a book shelf next to the bed—or even behind it—conveys the sense that something of great force and much weight, with sharp corners and edges, can fall onto the sleeping person.

The situation is completely different in office rooms. Here you can collect an infinite abundance of books (as long as they are placed in rows and not piled on top of each other in a disorderly way). However, don't forget to leave enough free space in the room so that the path of creativity and inspiration is not blocked.

Anyone who reads needs good lighting (see page15) and the zone in which the room is located naturally plays a substantial role (see Pa Kua, page 9).

Fragrances

Our perceptions are guided by our six senses (in addition to our classic five senses, a central function is assumed by the intuition, which is also called the inner voice) and one of these is the sense of smell. It exerts an extremely strong influence on our well-being. If we are hungry, the fragrances from the kitchen are heavenly. But if we are full, the smell of food begins to bother us. Our sense of smell reacts in the same sensitive and spontaneous manner to a bathroom.

The three main sources of chi energy are warmth, light, and fresh air. If we air on a regular basis, we can actively improve the quality of the oxygen and freshness of the air. This has a very positive effect on us.

However, we can do more than just renew our air. We can also improve it to achieve the quality that we like to smell. Essential oils, diffusers, incense, and artificially made fragrance stones are remedies for this purpose. Even cleaning agents contain olfactory substances so that everything appears to be clean, fresh, and light. In the automotive industry, specialists are consulted to make new cars smell like leather, luxury, something new, and natural materials as long as possible—rather than smelling of rubber and glue.

In feng shui, it is very important to observe that every room requires a different fragrance quality. While strong perfuming may be absolutely sensible in the bathroom, it is preferable for the kitchen to smell neutral. The living room is subject to the individual needs of its occupants. Some people like a stronger

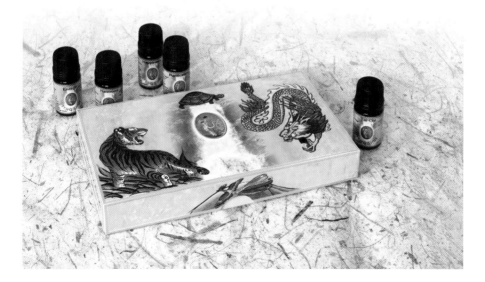

fragrance, while others are more sensitive and prefer a minimum of additional smells in a room. A sparing use of fragrances is also recommended for the bedroom. However, a sick room can experience a completely rejuvenating and beneficial effect through the application of oils. In the relationship and the family, the minimum tolerance for fragrances and necessary respect for how all occupants react to them should be observed. There are homes that always "smell like a woman." Then it's no surprise that the man no longer feels at home at some point. He first distances himself emotionally from his partner and then removes his entire self from the situation.

Since dried flowers embody something lifeless and dead, dried and perfumed flowers are absolutely unsuitable according to the teachings of feng shui. Logically speaking, these are not exactly in the appropriate state for awakening a room.

Angels

In China, there are no angels in the way that we know them. As a result, you will hardly find an angel figure with an Asiatic face. Our angels, guardian angels, are there for us in all of life's situations. The Chinese guardian angels have divided up their tasks among themselves: the dragon, the tiger, the tortoise, frogs, gnomes, stones, lions, jade disks, and many other entities have assumed one portion of a guardian angel's functions.

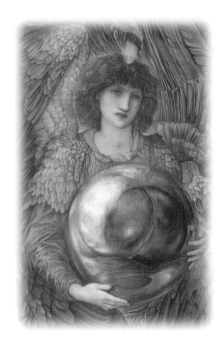

Even if angels have no "official" place in a book about Chinese balancing tools, they are still an important portion of our own culture and the most important heavenly helpers for us in the West. It is also interesting to note that "our" guardian angels with Western faces have experienced quite a boom in Hong Kong during the past few years. Many angels (with slender, masculine bodies) can also be found in the Thai culture.

The best location for all heavenly helpers as friends is Zone 6, but a guardian angel can never be in the wrong place. Anyone having money problems can also place a heavenly friend in Zone 4. A path in life (Zone 1) protected by angels should not be scorned and love (Zone 4) can also be entrusted to the protection of the angels. When you place an angel (or more than one), be sure that the surrounding area and the ceiling also radiates a slightly heavenly character. A light and airy effect should be created.

Windows

When Windows Face Each Other

Windows, as well as doors, are openings within the rooms that directly connect us with the good power of the sun's light and/or enable us to enter and leave a room. The first response to this idea is that a room should have as many windows as possible (like a winter garden) seems quite logical. However, an additional factor must be considered: the flow of energy. If two windows face each other, energy will cross-circulate between them. The best way to recognize these energy paths is when we open both windows while the wind is blowing outside. One of the windows (or even a door) will slam with such a loud bang that we are terribly startled.

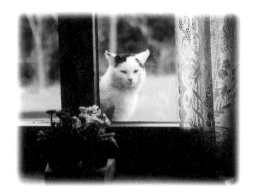

There are various possibilities for alleviating this cross-circulation of energy. The simplest variation for doors and windows that face each other is naturally to make one of the windows or one door (when there are several) inactive. Living rooms or kitchens can often be entered from two sides, whereby one of the doors could often be called "completely superfluous." It is much more sensible to turn a door into a wall and close it off with furniture than to "break up" the wall and lose the space. Even a kitchen cabinet, bookcase, corner bench, or sofa could find a good place there. However, a more specific method would be to deactivate a window by closing the shutters. If a door and a window face each other, go ahead and keep the window closed with the shutter during the day and night if the room has one or several other windows.

The complete closing of a window does not always simultaneously improve the quality of life within a room: the room may also become gloomy and dreary when a window is missing. However, there is another solution so that the occupants are not forced to constantly live in this cross-circulation of energy: dragon tears. With their enormous power, they block the direct path of the energy and divert its flow to all of the four walls or directions (also see pg. 46).

However, if a room has only one window and one door, nothing can be deactivated since the sense of well-being in it would only deteriorate as a result. Once again, there are naturally several possibilities for changing and improving it according to your needs. In a child's room, it actually isn't a problem if the door and window face each other as long as the child is small. When children go to bed, the window shutters are closed and the energy does not flow across them while they sleep. When children play, they are usually on the floor. However, the lower edge of a window usually begins at a height of 28 to 36 inches. Although the children may feel the energy circulating above their heads, they are not directly in the line of the flow. Light and colorful wind chimes and mobiles fit into any child's room and can calm this flow of energy between the door and the window.

When Windows Receive Too Little Sunlight

The north side of a house is naturally less indulged by the sun than the south side. Consequently, the sun can shine as much as it likes and the windows can be as large as possible but the room will only be warmed for a short time in the morning by the sun—or not at all. When houses are built very close together, it is only possible for the sunbeams to reach certain windows for a very short amount of time. In large cities, unfortunately, the upper stories often receive a lot of sunlight while the ground floor can only enjoy the sun for a short time because the neighboring house blocks and absorbs the sun's rays. You can capture the sunbeams with rainbow crystals. You can angle a little mirror on the windowsill so that the sun's energy comes into the depths of the room.

When There Are No Windows

Numerous apartments and houses have a room without windows. This is usually a little storeroom, toilet, or bathroom. The good energy of the sun has no possibility of touching and brightening the room in this situation. So the energy remains stuck in the room, becomes old, spent, and negative. In bathrooms and toilets that were built without a window, there is usually a ventilation system to provide for an exchange of the air. However, the missing feeling of space and light naturally cannot be created by even the best ventilation system since this isn't its purpose. Yet, there is a little trick for changing and alleviating this deficiency, which we clearly feel: we simulate a window in one wall.

The following materials are required for this purpose: a poster, a window frame, some glue, and a hanger. In order to make the illusion perfect, the most important factor is that the motif on the picture must naturally be appropriate. A landscape, a meadow, birds in the trees, or flowers could also be the view from

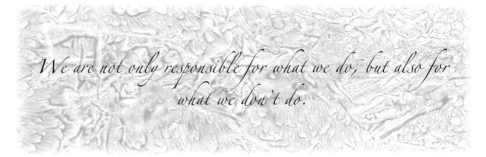

We are not only responsible for what we do, but also for what we don't do.

a window in reality. However, flowers in a vase are very inappropriate since flowers do not grow in vases anywhere outside when we look through a real window. There are also posters and pictures that show the view from a window and illustrate the entire frame or a slightly opened window (with the landscape behind it, of course). You can find window frames at a second-hand shop. When houses are renovated, old window frames are sometimes piled up in front of the building.

You can naturally also buy a window frame from a window company, but the price will definitely be somewhat higher. If you want to make the illusion perfect, a two-part window that closes in the middle and also contains window glass is the ideal solution. But the frame and the handle on the window that allow it to be opened are sufficient. In any case, it is very important to cover up the title of the picture. The name of the distributor and artist is usually printed in the lower right corner. Something like this naturally does not correspond in any way with the "natural view" through the window and must be covered up by the frame. If the hanger is installed in a somewhat discreet way, the perfect illusion of a window is created. Together with ventilation in the bathroom, this creates the feeling of fresh air and sunshine brightening the room.

Pets

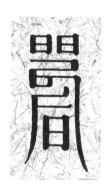

Pets are cheerful representatives of good energy. The more personality and character they possess, the greater their chi energy. The biggest carriers of constructive and strengthening energy are dogs and cats, followed by guinea pigs, hamsters, birds, turtles, and other small animals. Horses are not considered pets since they are too large.

Dogs

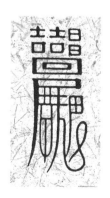

Dogs are said to be man's best friend and this is certainly true as long as the owner does not mistreat the animal companion. Dogs are infinitely loyal and it is their nature to protect their humans, above all from strangers and harm. Depending on their breed, dogs have various talents and preferences. Thanks to their ability to learn, they can be employed in the profession of rescuing humans, guarding herds of sheep, or protecting people and property. Man's best friend is associated with the element of earth and is therefore strengthened by the element of fire. Training and learning corresponds 100 percent to the fire element, which means that dogs enjoy learning new things.

However, not every dog owner wants to master more advanced tasks with an animal since most people just want a normal four-legged friend that wags, barks, and is content. So if a dog does not receive the element of fire that strengthens it through mental training, it can also achieve its necessary "fire portion" through the color red. The color red inside of its collar or its sleeping area or the pointy form of the doghouse roof—all of this can be selected in keeping with the element of fire.

Cats

Cats like to be on their own and love freedom and independence. They like to have their way and assert themselves. Just like they slink through the neighborhood for hours and are conspicuous in their absence, they can ensnare their human being in a cuddly and affectionate way. In feng shui, cats correspond with the element of metal. They are the messengers of the gods and accompany the immortals, the sorcerers, and the God of Wealth. (We could almost think that they slink around at the request of the gods.) They protect the wealth that slumbers in the element of earth and are therefore strengthened by all yellow and brown tones. Because cats can see at night, they belong to the yin energy. However, the Chinese equate them with the three unreasonable yang animals during the mating season because of how they scream when they live out their instincts.

Birds

To the Chinese, singing birds mean good luck. Anyone accompanied by a bird in a little bamboo cage takes good luck along on the path. Since the Chinese like to gamble and games of chance are dependent upon luck, as the name implies, it is obvious that a gambler brings his bird with him. However, singing birds in the outdoors also mean good luck. Incidentally, people in China show off the beauty and singing abilities of their birds in exactly the same way as people in the West show off their cars.

In the Western world, the birds stay at home in their cages and are sometimes also allowed freedom of movement within the home since they tend to be part of the family. Animal companions are usually seen as fellow residents, which is a good idea.

Fish

Fish are always a symbol of wealth and abundance in China and Japan. Chinese goldfish cannot be compared with their Western counterparts since they are quite fat and round, sometimes growing to a size of 12 inches. Top prices are paid for these fish, depending upon their color. If a goldfish has the white circle of the nation's flag in Japan, it is worth a fortune.

Little Rodents

Guinea pigs and hamsters are very popular pets for children. For the Chinese, the little fur-bearing animals (including mice and rats) are always a symbol of charm and mental agility. They are associated with the element of water since they love togetherness and communication. The element of metal gives them power and strength. You can make the little rodents very happy with gray or white boxes and cages, as well as furnishings made of metal.

Here are a few special cases:

Spiders

Most of us usually don't think of spiders as desirable pets, yet they still find their way into our apartments and houses time and again. There is a German saying that spiders "only live in good houses." In China, a spider descending on a thread from its web is seen as a messenger of the heavens that wants to bring joy to humanity. Even if you don't want to give your personal house spider "long-term asylum," you can help it move but allow this "messenger of the heavens" to stay alive.

Bats

Bats are a traditional Chinese symbol of good luck since the Chinese word for both luck and bat are spoken as FU. One legend tells how the bat did not appear for the birthday of the phoenix or the unicorn, telling them both that it is neither bird nor quadruped. When the truth was exposed, all of the animals were surprised at the craftiness of the bat. Since then, it has been a symbol for sly actions.

Guests and Visitors from the Animal World

Cats, birds, and even hedgehogs meet in some gardens because they either feel extremely good there or someone provides for them. A little ceramic bowl can become a meeting place for birds so they can bathe here after it has rained. A little covered bird table can be a very important address for birds during a severe winter.

Music

When energy is heard, it is expressed as tones. The music that appeals to us sometimes varies considerably, and we also have greatly differing preferences in terms of the volume. At a very early point in time, the Chinese determined that certain tones, melodies, rhythms, and volumes influence our organs and cleanse our meridians so that qi energy can flow freely. As a result, a type of "therapeutic-medicinal music" was created that is now called Feng Shui Music or Five Element Music. This music is capable to cause subtle healing effects and to awaken unexpected powerful energies.

Another form of music is silence. It is a great, powerful source of energy that rightfully has a place in all of the renowned writings.

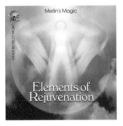

Merlin's Magic
Elements of Rejuvenation
–Qi Gong Energy Healing–
Inner Worlds Music
CD 41094 · ISBN: 0-910261-43-1

Acknowledgments

I would like to heartily thank all of these individuals and companies for their spontaneity and helpfulness in providing support for this book with feng shui articles, slides, and Chinese objects of good fortune.

Luo Pan (page 62): Mr. Marc Haeberin—thanks again for the absolutely wonderful assistance.

Various Chinese objects of good fortune: Thank you so much to Trinh Truong, who took down his very personal symbols of good luck and decorative articles in his store to give them to me for this book.

Calligraphies: were drawn by the grand master Samuel Kwok, to whom I am thankful from the depths of my heart. An infinite thank-you to the grand master Kwok, who transformed my kitchen into a magical room of calligraphy and whose energy and strength has been perceptible in his characters since the creation of the pictures.

Mobiles: Dear Ms. Kiener, thank you so much for all your efforts and the beautiful mobiles that are your very own creations.

Incense (page 69), **feng shui gift sets** (page 85), **and room fountains** (page 29): I thank PRIMAVERA LIFE GmbH, for the permission to print their wonderful product photos.

When you came into the world, you cried
and everyone around you was delighted
Live so that when you leave the world
Everyone will cry
And you alone will smile.
—*Chinese saying*—

Epilog

This book has come to an end. The more I become involved with balancing tools, the better I understand the phrase and life philosophy that my father taught me: "Live each day as if it were your last."

Good fortune also means being inwardly free, owing nothing to anyone—whether in material or emotional terms, as well as saying what we think, treating each other lovingly, and living the great values of tolerance, respect, and dignity. And so now I wish you, dear reader of this book, all the good fortune of this world.

Yours truly, Brigitte Gaertner

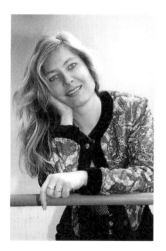

About the Author

Lao-tse gave her wings and a Tibetan monk prepared the landing field. The result: With her head in the clouds, Brigitte Gaertner has her feet on the ground. A deep rootedness in Asian culture, meditation, aesthetics, and the Five Elements are part of the author's life. She is involved in the book-trade and holds pendulum seminars, as well as offering feng shui consultations oriented toward harmony and good experiences.

Titles Released by LOTUS PRESS • SHANGRI-LA

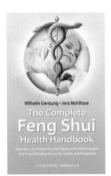

Wilhelm Gerstung · Jens Mehlhase
The Complete Feng Shui Health Handbook
How You Can Protect Yourself Against Harmful Energies and Create Positive Forces for Health and Prosperity
This fascinating handbook provides many graphics and practical information, which help design every home in such a way that it becomes a source of energy. The authors integrate their many years of research and extensive knowledge of energies in the home and sleeping area, with the Western science of underground watercourses and grids.

224 pages · $16.95 · ISBN 0914955-60-8

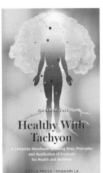

Andreas Jell
Healthy with Tachyon
A Complete Handbook Including Basic Principles and Application of Products for Health and Wellness
A completely new chapter of human history has begun with the possibility of directly applying tachyon energy for healing and development. Today, you can directly strengthen your powers of self-healing by using tachyonized materials. These powers will then organize perfect healing and development (anti-entropy) through their own dynamic.

144 pages · $12.95 · ISBN 0-914955-58-6

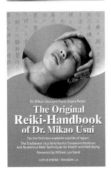

Dr. Mikao Usui and Frank Arjava Petter
The Original Reiki Handbook of Dr. Mikao Usui
The Traditional Usui Reiki Ryoho Treatment Positions and Numerous Reiki Techniques for Health and Well-Being
For the first time available outside of Japan. The original hand positions and healing techniques from Dr. Usui's handbook have been listed in detail, making it a valuable reference work for anyone who practices Reiki. Whether you are an initiate or a master, if you practice Reiki you can expand your knowledge dramatically as you follow in the footsteps of a great healer.

80 pages ·100 photos · $14.95 · ISBN 0-914955-57-8

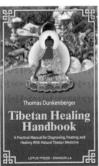

Thomas Dunkenberger
Tibetan Healing Handbook
A Practical Manual for Diagnosing, Treating, and Healing with Natural Tibetan Medicine
The author describes the entire spectrum of application possibilities for Tibetan medicine and its use for treatment purposes. At the same time, he provides information about holistic remedies so that you can take action to restore your inner harmony and health. This practical step-by-step manual offers you the benefits of diagnosing, treating, and healing with natural Tibetan medicine.

240 pages · $15.95 · ISBN 0-914955-66-7

INNER WORLDS MUSIC FOR RELAXATION AND ENERGIZATION

Elements of Rejuvenation
Merlin's Magic
A New Album for Invigorating Your Universal Qi and Essence
This music has been composed especially for qi gong, and is also suitable for yoga and t'ai chi. The uplifting melodies flow smoothly in resonance with subtle qi movements and awaken energies that are unexpectedly powerful. Listening to these exceptional qi sounds will allow you to become more deeply in touch with the universal life energy and heal yourself.
$17.95 CD 0-910261-43-1 · INNER WORLDS MUSIC

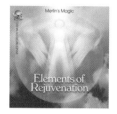

Chakra Meditation "Audio"
Merlin's Magic · Sharamon, Baginski
Presents an acoustic journey through the energy centres. As you softly move through each chakra, you will be immersed into the universal life force, enhancing your receptivity for deep feelings, experiencing a special bond with the creation as a whole and resonating with your inner power in a blissful state of perfect contentment.
$17.95 CD 0-910261-57-1 · $10.95 CA 0-910261-80-6 · INNER WORLDS MUSIC

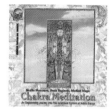

Reiki: Light Touch
Merlin's Magic
This beautiful, serenely blissful instrumental music is a true gift for healing and happiness. Its soothing sounds and caressing vibrations are wonderful for many different forms of bodywork, energy balancing, meditating, or just relaxing. Guitar combined with keyboards, violin, viola, and deeply resonant Tibetan bells create the relaxing sound of Light Touch.
$17.95 CD 0-910261-85-7 · $10.95 CA 0-910261-79-2 · INNER WORLDS MUSIC

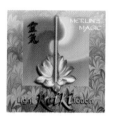

Healing Harmony—The Best of Merlin's Magic
Merlin's Magic
Merlin's Magic is a best-seller in the field of healing and relaxing music. Now they present a wonderful compilation of selections from their four previous albums, plus two new compositions. Whether you want to relax, or to use music as a therapeutic background for massage, Reiki or bodywork, this recording will delight you!
$17.95 CD 0-910261-50-4 · $10.95 CA 0-910261-48-2 · INNER WORLDS MUSIC

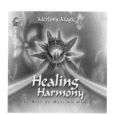

Waves of Love—A Must for Every Saxophone Lover
Eden River
Headed by Andreas Mock and featuring saxophonist Lee Mayall, this album makes you feel like lying in the arms of your beloved one, makes you feel one with eternal love of the universe. Music for the heart, accompanied by the dance of a saxophone, as it has never heard before. Flute, piano, and violin join in a choreography of sweeping emotions.
$17.95 CD 0-910261-51-2 · INNER WORLDS MUSIC

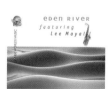

For information and additional recordings:
INNER WORLDS MUSIC · P.O. Box 325 · Twin Lakes · WI 53181· USA · (800) 444-9678

Herbs and other natural health products and information are often available at natural food stores or metaphysical bookstores. If you cannot find what you need locally, you can contact one of the following sources of supply.

Sources of Supply:

The following companies have an extensive selection of useful products and a long track-record of fulfillment. They have natural body care, aromatherapy, flower essences, crystals and tumbled stones, homeopathy, herbal products, vitamins and supplements, videos, books, audio tapes, candles, incense and bulk herbs, teas, massage tools and products and numerous alternative health items across a wide range of categories.

WHOLESALE:

Wholesale suppliers sell to stores and practitioners, not to individual consumers buying for their own personal use. Individual consumers should contact the RETAIL supplier listed below. Wholesale accounts should contact with business name, resale number or practitioner license in order to obtain a wholesale catalog and set up an account.

Lotus Light Enterprises, Inc.

P. O. Box 1008
Silver Lake, WI 531 70 USA
262 889 8501 (phone)
262 889 8591 (fax)
800 548 3824 (toll free order line)

RETAIL:

Retail suppliers provide products by mail order direct to consumers for their personal use. Stores or practitioners should contact the wholesale supplier listed above.

Internatural

33719 116th Street
Twin Lakes, WI 53181 USA
800 643 4221 (toll free order line)
262 889 8581 office phone
WEB SITE: www.internatural.com

Web site includes an extensive annotated catalog of more than 7000 products that can be ordered "on line" for your convenience 24 hours a day, 7 days a week.